PSYCHO-MOTOR BEHAVIOR IN
EDUCATION AND SPORT

PSYCHO-MOTOR BEHAVIOR IN EDUCATION AND SPORT

~~~~~~~~~~ SELECTED PAPERS ~~~~~~~~~~

By

BRYANT J. CRATTY

University of California

Los Angeles, California

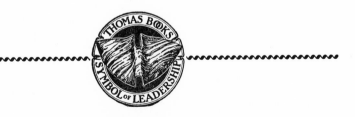

CHARLES C THOMAS · PUBLISHER

Springfield, Illinois, U.S.A.

Published and Distributed Throughout the World by
CHARLES C THOMAS • PUBLISHER
Bannerstone House
301-327 East Lawrence Avenue, Springfield, Illinois, U.S.A.

© 1974, by CHARLES C THOMAS • PUBLISHER
ISBN 0-398-03099-5
Library of Congress Catalog Card Number: 73 21972

Library of Congress Cataloging in Publication Data

Cratty, Bryant J
  Psycho-motor behavior in education and sport; selected papers.

  Bibliography: p.
  1. Perceptual-motor learning. 2. Motor learning. 3. Learning ability.
4. Physical education for children. I. Title. [DNLM: 1. Motor activity. 2.
Psychology, Educational. 3. Sports. QT260 C896p 1974]
LB1067.C73   370.15′2   73–21972
ISBN 0–398–03099–5

Printed in the United States of America
K-8

ACKNOWLEDGMENTS

DURING THE PAST seven or eight years I have been frequently the guest of educational institutions, parent organizations, institutes serving atypical children and youth, as well as of international symposia engaged in scholarly discourse about various aspects of psycho-motor activity. I have on two other occasions during this period published papers, and essays which have been delivered during these various meetings, symposia, workshops and lectures. The papers within this monograph represent the third collection of these reports, together with summaries of research we have carried out at UCLA, between the years 1970 to 1973.

Within this same period of time I have been supported in my work in the Perceptual-Motor Learning Laboratory by the U.S. Department of Education's Bureau of Education for the Handicapped, by travel and research grants from UCLA's Academic Senate, by travel grants from the University of Brussels, and from the government of Spain. To these governments and agencies I would like to give my thanks. The work on dynamic visual acuity was assisted by the Institute for Transportation and Traffic Engineering here at UCLA, and by their research psychologist, Dr. Albert Burg. Mr. Reinhard Bergel and Mr. Erwin Apitzsch assisted in the collection of data in that same investigation. Mr. Lloyd Percival, director of the Fitness Institute at Toronto, Canada provided the impetus for two papers dealing with athletics, due to his sponsorship of the Symposium on the Art and Science of Coaching in 1971. Dr. Marcel Hebbelink, from the University of Brussels was my host at the World Federation of

Physical Education Conference in 1973, while Dr. Jose Cagigal was also a gracious host to me the same year, at the 3rd International Congress of Sports Psychology in Madrid. Papers from both of these meetings are contained in this publication. Mr. Robert Bonds collected data for the comparative study of the physical abilities of Afro-American and Chicano and Anglo children which is found in the following pages.

Mrs. Sally Cooper was my hostess in Atlanta, Georgia in the summer of 1973, and the paper dealing with a model for the development of the body image reflects this visit. The Publication Committee of the California Association for Neurologically Handicapped Children kindly permitted me to reprint the "Answers to Questions Parents Ask," while the paper dealing with the effects of learning games upon academic abilities of children is the result of research with which I was assisted by Sisters Margaret Mary Martin, O.S.F., M.A. and Mark Szczepanik, O.S.F., B.S. from 1967–1971.

To all the aforementioned ladies and gentlemen I would like to express my thanks. Misses Diane Birnbaum and Sara Solberg prepared the final manuscript; thus I am grateful to them also.

BJC

CONTENTS

Part IV
The Athlete: Psychological Considerations

PSYCHO-MOTOR BEHAVIOR IN EDUCATION AND SPORT

PART I

INTELLIGENCE IN EDUCATION
SPORT AND
PHYSICAL EDUCATION

INTELLECTUAL ATTRIBUTES
AND SPORTS PERFORMANCE*

A THLETES IN COMPETITION, as well as children in physical education classes, are often treated by their mentors as though
they were simplistic, muscular servo-mechanisms. Much of the
literature in physical education and sports teaching concentrates
upon what the trainer, coach, and/or instructor will do for, or to,
athletes, while still other literature in sport psychology has con-
centrated upon what one might resort to if the athlete does not
prove flexible and does not bend effortlessly to the tutoring
offered him.

In contrast to this often rather mechanistic approach to
eliciting superior sports performance is a large volume of literature concentrating upon the complex nature of human intelligence. Such profound questions as the relative influence of nature
and nurture upon the development of the mind may be traced
from the earliest writings of the Greeks and Romans through
the emergence of the first organized approaches to the measurement of intelligence, to the more sophisticated models of the
intellect emerging in the last two decades.†

Only seldom, however, has there been even a superficial wedding of information about human intelligence and various parameters of athletic endeavor. Thorpe and West, for example,
have published some provocative pilot efforts concerning the
intellectual precursors to what they term "game sense." [9] At least

---

* Speech for the 3rd International Congress of Sports Psychology, Madrid, Spain,
June 25–29, 1973.

† A review of the history of intelligence testing may be found in Chapter 1, "Historical Trends," in B. J. Cratty, *Physical Expressions of Intelligence* (Englewood
Cliffs, Prentice-Hall, Inc., 1972).

four other researchers argue somewhat vaguely for the importance of "abstract reasoning ability" [6,7,8] and "intellectual aspiration" in the performance of superior athletes.

Even a cursory look at research about human intelligence
carried out since World War II, however, points to the re-
markable complexity of the concept and the diffusion and relative independence of various intellectual functions. Guilford,
for example, in his "Structure of the Intellect" model, suggests
that there are more than eighty independent abilities, based upon
the interactions of three major dimensions. These dimensions
include: operations or the levels of functioning including
memory, evaluation, convergent production (perceiving all possibilities), divergent production (arriving at best answers, solutions), and cognition. The second dimension is content and includes the figural, the symbolic (letters, numbers), the semantic
(words) and finally the behavioral (social behaviors for the
most part). Guilford names as "products" the outcome of intelligent behaviors and includes classes, relations, systems, trans-
formation, and forming implications.[5]

There are numerous other typologies of intellectual behavior
including those by Gagne [4] and Bloom,[1] which do not rest upon
as much data as does Guilford's and at the same time are simpler
to comprehend.

Despite the lack of data dealing in precise ways with mental-
motor relationships within an athletic context, sports psychologists on both sides of the Atlantic and Pacific Oceans have written at various times about the influence of mental practice upon
skill attainment, of "ideomotor training" [10] and about the importance of instilling in superior athletes a firm grasp of scientific
principles underlying the performance of their sport. Workshops
in various parts of the world have attempted at various times to
impart knowledge about physiology, sociology, and psychology
as they pertain to athletic endeavor with both athletes and
coaches taking part. However, if sports scientists from various
of the disciplines truly hold the philosophical belief that man is
a thinking animal as well as a performing one, it should then
follow that attempting to synthesize and analyze the interactions
of various aspects of sports performance and the multidimen-

sional nature of intelligent behavior is a productive undertaking.

In an effort to somehow bring some order to the apparent chaos, which could result from an unorganized look at these two dimensions of human behavior, the following model has been developed. Its purpose is to delineate some of the major areas for study and scientific exploration; at the same time the model suggests that certain types of philosophically based judgments may at times interact with some of the more pragmatic considerations.

Essentially, the model contains three major axes, with one of these fragmented in turn into two parts. The first dimension, but not necessarily the most important, is one which suggests that a continuum, or scale, exists, upon which someone must decide just *whose* intellect shall predominate, who shall be responsible for making judgments based upon intellectual competencies: the coach or his athlete. At the same time, since this dimension is in truth a flexible scale, it often may be appropriate that neither the mind of the coach nor that of the athlete should dominate, but that cooperative decisions should be made concerning various aspects of training and game performance. It is likely that during the career of an athlete he will find himself operating, or forced to operate along various parts of the scale. During his early career he may be content to depend entirely upon the judgment of his coach, while later he may rightfully make an increasing number of the decisions influencing his athletic welfare. It is obvious that not only will the level of intellectual abilities both athlete and coach bring to a situation influence where along this scale both will operate, but that critical personality qualities including authoritarianism, succor and dependency in both coach and participant will influence the manner in which each will accept the decisions of the other.

The second dimension shown is a temporal one, and this in turn has been fragmented into two parts, one indicating short-term career of both coach and athlete. Within the shorter of the two temporal dimensions are considerations as to when certain types of intellectual decisions are necessary; for example, there may be sports in which precompetition training decisions are more important than are those confronting a swimmer or runner during the time he actually participates. On the other hand, tactical decisions during a team game may be as important as those governing training sessions.

The second, long-term, temporal dimension reflects the career of coach or athlete and suggests that the quality and/or quantity of intellectual involvement and intelligent decision-making may vary as both coach and athlete gain experience and acquire increased amounts of information about the sport in which both are interested. The fledgling athlete may not be qualified and may be reluctant to offer intellectual input; whereas the more seasoned performer may have become both qualified and useful as a thinker about the sport in which he is participating. Moreover the athlete or coach at career's end may also change his inclinations about inserting thoughts into an action situation.

The final, primary dimension depicted in the model is one which suggests that there are several levels of intellectual functioning. For clarity, only five have been included. It should not be inferred, upon inspecting the diagram, that a given decision about a sport involves only a single intellectual dimension. For example, a coach or athlete, when searching for an appropriate tactical decision in a soccer game, will usually engage first in divergent production and memory (innumerating mentally and/or verbally *all* the possibilities) and then secondly *evaluate* which of those retrieved from his memory is the most desirable and best one to use. Naturally, the speed with which these processes are engaged in is often critical in eliciting a positive outcome. Within this dimension it is believed that the most helpful type of intellectual behavior in which both athlete and coach may engage may be intellectual flexibility, the willingness to cast off inappropriate but previously employed methods, strategies, and/or skills. Within this same component is the quality of being able to adopt old principles in new ways and of formulating new principles and strategies to meet new and, at times, unexpected situations, events, and conditions.

An Overview

In these few minutes I have attempted to paint, in rather broad strokes, my concepts of a problem area which I believe is

**A MODEL FOR THE STUDY OF INTELLIGENT BEHAVIORS IN
ATHLETICS**

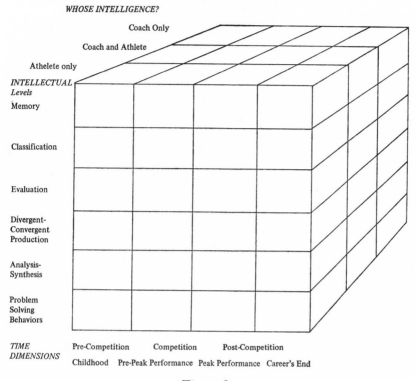

Figure 1.

tremendously complex. There are numerous subproblems, which
hopefully will be explored both scientifically and philosophically
by some of those in attendance, and which are beginning to
elicit interest in general education as well as in sports education
around the world.

Man has been described by some naturalists and philosophers
as the only "thinking animal"—a debatable distinction upon inspecting apparently intelligent behaviors of even some of our
more distant relatives on the phylogenic scale. At the same time
it is believed that man is the only animal who devoted time and
effort to *thinking about thinking,* a fruitful process and one
which, it is hoped, received impetus here.

BIBLIOGRAPHY

1. Bloom, Benjamin (Ed.): *Taxonomy of Educational Objectives, Handbook I Cognitive Domain.* New York, McKay, 1956.
2. Cratty, B. J.: *Psychology in Contemporary Sport.* Englewood Cliffs, P-H, 1973.
3. ———: *Physical Expressions of Intelligence.* Englewood Cliffs, P-H, 1972.
4. Gagne, R. W.: *The Conditions of Learning.* New York: HR&W, 1965.
5. Guilford, J. P.: *The Nature of Human Intelligence.* New York, McGraw, 1967.
6. Kane, John: Personality and Physical Abilities. In Kenyon, Gerald S. (Ed.): *Contemporary Psychology of Sport.* Chicago, Athletic Institute, 1970.
7. Ogilvie, Bruce: Psychological consistencies within high level competitors. In *JAMA* Special Olympic Year Edition, September–October, 1968, vol. XXIV.
8. Rushall, Brent: An evaluation of the relationship between personality and physical performance categories. In Kenyon, Gerald S. (Ed.): *Contemporary Psychology of Sport,* Chicago, Athletic Institute, 1970.
9. Thorpe, JoAnne and West, Charlotte: Game sense and intelligence. *Percept Mot Skills,* 29:326, 1969.
10. Vanek, Miroslav and Cratty, B. J.: *Psychology and the Superior Athlete.* New York, Macmillan, 1969.

FREEDOM OF THE INTELLECT:

A RESOLUTION OF FORCES*

∿∿∿

EDUCATIONAL PHILOSOPHERS from Plato, and Seneca to John Guilford, and Jerome Bruner, have speculated about the nature of the human intellect. And while their techniques, starting points, and conclusions differ widely, common to those of their writings is the implication that the maturing child should somehow be encouraged to think for himself. The youth, these writers seem to infer, should be somehow released from constraints and be encouraged to explore, speculate, to arrive at wrong as well as correct conclusions and to somehow become a creative adult. These same writers and philosophers are hardly in agreement, however, as to just how these goals may be achieved in specific and operational ways.

Within recent literature there seem to be two threads which if somehow reconciled, could lead to the productive outcomes outlined by the aforementioned writers. One of these inferences, found primarily in the work of Guilford, Gagné, and Bloom, suggests that intellectual tasks may be arranged in a hierarchical order, from relatively simple (usually memory) tasks, to those which are more difficult, and include problem solving, the formulation and transference of principles and similar processes and operations. These same writers and researchers furthermore suggest that school personnel make certain that they insert experiences which tend to tax children and youth at all points along their intellectual continuum or taxonomy. At the same time it is not often clear just what kinds of operations are likely to plug

---

* Prepared for the Special Education Department, University of Hawaii's Symposium on Learning and Motor Learning, October 5, 1973.

children into certain kinds of problem-solving and intellectual operations, upon consulting these same writings.

The second thread has been expounded by Bruner, and in rather operational terms by Mosston. These individuals suggest that the production of a creative intellect unhampered by the constraints of undue conformity, may evolve if the teacher participates in a gradual and appropriate shift of decisions from her (and from the school hierarchy) to the students, when the latter seem capable of accepting the decisions while maintaining some kind of teacher-student structure.

This general approach has been further analyzed by Mosston in two publications, and is based upon the premise that common to all educational programs and processes is the need to make decisions. Mosston would then have the teacher and students compile a list of the types of decisions which might be adopted by either the authority figure or the subordinates. This list, from the temporal standpoint Mosston suggests, may be divided into three main subdivisions: decisions made prior to the lesson, decisions occurring during the lesson, and post-lesson decisions (these latter consisting for the most part of evaluative efforts).

Mosston further proposes that teaching behavior may be placed on a continuum, "From Command to Discovery," ranging from behaviors reflecting an authoritative orientation on the part of the instructor in which he or she makes all decisions, and the students may only passively respond, to one in which most of the planning and evaluative decisions have been transferred to the students.*

In demonstrations, and in written lessons Mosston has explored several phenomena related to his schema including (a) the difficulty passive students may have in accepting decisions extended to them, (b) the difficulties authoritarian teachers may

---

* Although proponents of this general approach deny their own authoritarian tendencies, it seems to this writer that both their writings and lectures reflect a dogmatism relative to the suggestion that their schema is the only logical one to adopt; while within the methodology one catches glimpses of what could be construed as covert manipulations by instructors as they encourage "guided" discovery . . . or "correct principles" . . . While furthermore it is apparent that the teacher in rather arbitrary ways is deciding just when, and what decisions should be shifted to her or his charges.

have in truly extending important decisions to their students, and (c) behaviors related to what Mosston has described as "breaking" the cognitive barrier, on the part of students.

Like Festinger and others, Mosston supports the premise that learning to think independently is at times somewhat painful, and refers frequently in his work to the importance of creating "cognitive dissonance" defined as a period of struggle or conflict which is important to create within the teaching-learning environment—a conundrum which when resolved will likely result in a more enlightened student, one who becomes more able to think for himself or herself.

Others, including Bloom and Gagné, have produced typologies containing groups or classifications of intellectual processes, which seem to be arranged in hierarchical orders which are dependent upon the apparent difficulty of the operation engaged in by the thinker. Bloom's six levels consist of knowledge (simple recall of facts), comprehension (the lowest form of understanding), application (the use of abstractions in specific situations); and in addition his scale ascends intellectually to analysis (breaking down information into parts in order to form clearer associations between ideas or concepts), synthesis (evolving new structures or patterns not formerly present), and finally evaluation, (judgments made about materials and methods, both quantitative and qualitative based upon criteria evolved by others or by the learner himself).

Gagné arranges the levels within his hierarchy also from the simple to the complex, reflecting the orientation of a Skinnerian learning theorist: These seven levels consist of response differentiation (simply copying a stimulus via exact replication), association (responding with an answer which may not be the exact stimulus presented, but is the only answer possible under the conditions presented), multiple discrimination (selection of a correct response when presented with two or more potentially confusing stimuli), behavior chains (recalling a chain of stimuli logically attached to one presented, i.e. reciting a poem), and class concepts (the forming of discriminations based upon their general characteristics, rather than upon specific ones). Gagné's hierarchy finishes with two additional processes or operations including principles (application of a single rule within several situations), and "problem-solving strategies" (the discovery of principles for solving a series of novel situations, providing mediating responses in stimulus-response situations to meet specified goals).

Although space does not permit an even partial exposure of Guilford's complex "Model of the Intellect" suffice to say that it is more expansive than the more laminated type of models outlined by Gagné and Bloom. Guilford suggests that the human intellectual processes may be only explained with reference to three major dimensions termed (a) "operations" (composed of five subareas), (b) "products" (consisting of six subcomponents, covering the outcomes of intellectual endeavors), and finally (c) "content," comprising the "stuff" which is thought about, and including four different subcomponents. It is not clear to this writer whether Guilford believes that certain operations, the manipulation of specific products, and/or the production of specific outcomes are considered harder than others. At the same time explicit in Guilford's writings is the suggestion that classroom teachers operationalize their presentations so as to cover the broad spectrum of intellectual behaviors suggested by his model.

A Resolution of Forces

Thus two general approaches have been briefly outlined: (a) one which suggests that transferring decision-making to the learner, is the most expedient method of his promoting intellectual involvement, and (b) a second which suggests that indeed intellectual behaviors may be arranged from those which involve rather simple processes and operations to the more difficult, generally those in which the learner must produce new solutions, transfer principles and formulate and solve unique problems.

Upon consideration of these two threads I believe that the most productive strategy would be to resolve the two forces they represent—one a thrust for freedom, the second a thrust toward increased complexity and difficulty. That is, the learner must not simply be encouraged to adopt more and more decisions about content, evaluation, etc., within the educational setting;

A RESOLUTION OF FORCES IN EDUCATION

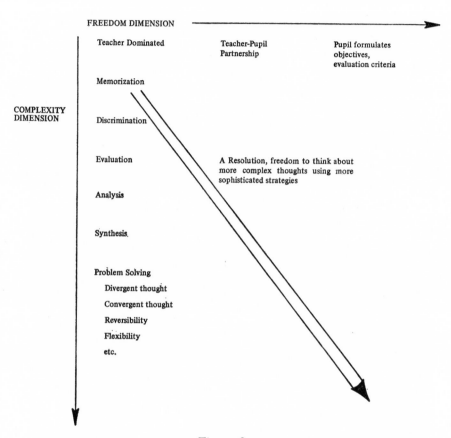

Figure 2.

or he may begin to engage in relatively meaningless endeavors, and remain submerged in trivia. On the other hand a curriculum in which, in authoritarian ways, the student is led toward increasingly difficult problems, again may do little to produce a truly creative thinker, one who feels free to err, to speculate and to produce new information, and strategies. Rather it is advanced that one must try to achieve freedom, in increasing amounts when the learner appears ready to accept it, and in subtle ways to lead (not manipulate) the learner to thinking about increasingly complex problems, content, and strategies for the solution of these problems. The teacher who tries to achieve a feeling of freedom to think, to be wrong, and to be different on the part of his students is indeed performing a noble service. But at times this service may lack depth, and may be intellectually shallow. However, the teacher who perceives, not only that students might be accorded increasing freedoms, but at the same time realizes that they may be exposed and encouraged to tax themselves as they are confronted with problems of increased significance, and complexity, would seem to be rendering her or his young charges an even greater service.

BIBLIOGRAPHY

1. Bloom, Benjamin S.: *Stability and Change in Human Characteristics.* New York, Wiley, 1964.
2. Bruner, Jerome (Ed.): *Learning About Learning.* U.S. Department of Health, Education and Welfare, Office of Education, Monograph 15, 1966.
3. Bruner, Jerome S.: The course of cognitive growth. *Am Psychol*, XXV: 1–15, January, 1964.
4. Bruner, Jerome S.: *Toward a Theory of Instruction.* Cambridge, Belknap Pr, Harvard U Pr, 1966.
5. Cratty, B. J.: *Human Behavior: Exploring Educational Processes.* Wolfe City, University Pr, 1972.
6. Cratty, B. J.: *Intelligence in Action.* Englewood Cliffs, P-H, 1973.
7. Cratty, B. J.: *Physical Expressions of Intelligence.* Englewood Cliffs, P-H, 1970, 1972.
8. Festinger, Leon: *The Theory of Cognitive Dissonance.* Evanston, Row, Peterson, 1957.
9. Gagné, Robert M.: *Learning and Individual Differences.* Columbus, Merrill, 1967.
10. Gagné, Robert M.: *The Conditions of Learning.* New York, HR&W, 1965.
11. Guilford, John P.: *Intelligence, Creativity and Their Intellectual Implications.* San Diego, Knapp, 1968.
12. Guilford, J. P.: *The Nature of Human Intelligence.* New York, McGraw, 1967.
13. Mosston, M.: *Teaching: From Command to Discovery.* Belmont, Wadsworth Pub, 1972.
14. Mosston, M.: *Teaching Physical Education.* Columbus, Merrill, 1967.
15. Popham, James W. and Baker, E. L.: *Systematic Instruction.* Englewood Cliffs, 1970.

CHAPTER 3

PHYSICAL CONTENT IN EDUCATIONAL PROGRAMS: ISSUES, CONUNDRUMS AND TRANSFER OF TRAINING*

EMPHASIS UPON ACTION within educational programs is not a new phenomenon. One may trace back emphases upon sensory-motor experiences within curricula for superior, normal, and less than normal youngsters by referring to early pedagogical writings.† The ancient Greeks held strongly to the inseparability of mind and body as they placed keen, intelligent faces atop their well-muscled statues. Pedagogical beginnings of sensory-motor experiences are seen in the writings of Renaissance educators of the young, normal child, as well as pedagogists interested in the abnormal youngster during this period of awakening. Itard, for example, is said to have employed sensory-motor experiences as part of the program he used to work with the legendary "Wild Boy of Aveyron"; later, the workbooks of Montessori contained innumerable types of motor experiences for young children, from those requiring balance, to games in which youngsters were asked to collect together, divide and count their fellow classmates in efforts to instill mathematical operations and concepts.[1]

---

* Prepared for a main lecture, in the Symposium on Transfer and Motor Learning, July 5–6, 1973, sponsored by the International Federation of Physical Education, held in Brussels, Belgium.

† A history of relationships between mental and motor components within educational programs and in testing strategies may be found in B. J. Cratty, *Physical Expressions of Intelligence*, Englewood Cliffs, Prentice-Hall, Inc., 1972.

The first experimental psychologists in continental Europe, as well as in England and the United States during the 1880's, began to explore what they termed the "faculties theory" of intelligence, by attempting to determine whether rather basic sensory, sensory-motor and kinesthetic measures were valid predictors of intelligence. Their efforts, coupled with the invention of techniques permitting correlation, proved that tests of reaction time, kinesthesis, and the like were not helpful predictors of intelligent behaviors which seemed to contribute to school success. However, one is still able to find sensory-motor components within contemporary tests of intelligence employed in most countries of the world.[1]

During the later 1940's in the United States, a text was published by Strauss and Lehtinen entitled *The Psychopathology and Education of the Brain-Injured Child* [12] in which a syndrome of behavior seen in confused, underachieving children was described, and included motor clumsiness. The group of symptoms also included hyperactivity, perceptual disturbances, as well as problems with classroom operations, including reading and writing. This book was soon followed by others in the early 1950's in which were proposed theories which rested upon the premise that "movement is the basis for the intelligent," and which expounded upon the rationale that not only were sound intellectual and perceptual functioning dependent upon good motor functioning, but that (a) if one was clumsy, perceptual difficulties including ineptitude in various academic skills were inevitable outcomes and (b) that to improve perceptual functioning and a variety of academic skills, one merely had to engage in a prescribed set of sensory-motor (or perceptual-motor) tasks.[9,10]

Practices arising from this type of widely expounded type of theory began to proliferate in the schools of the United States and in other countries of the world in the 1950's and particularly in the 1960's and 1970's. The theory was easy to understand, so that even the slightly trained could establish a sensory-motor program and monitor the efforts of children walking balance beams, touching balls swinging suspended from strings and the like.[10]

These programs evidenced many desirable, and at times undesirable, outcomes. For example, among the most desirable ones were the fact that some educators began to focus upon the more clumsy children in their midst, and at times the program of movement activities to which they were exposed truly helps them to improve. Children often ignored were given extra attention, while other children formerly blunted in their reading efforts by too many exposures to the printed page each week, were given respites in the form of jumping on trampolines, a study break which spaced the practice of reading in helpful ways and often resulted in improvement.

Less than desirable outcomes also accompanied what, at times, amounts to an hysterical adherence to various of the programs. For example, many parents became convinced that simply applied, motor activities would indeed improve high level academic skills, and when this was not forthcoming, further frustrations for both child as well as parent transpired. Many educators and parents were indoctrinated in the assumptions that all clumsy children must have learning difficulties and that all well-coordinated children must be free of the same, assumptions which are not substantiated upon exposing children to comprehensive batteries of tests evaluating several aspects of intelligence, and academic skills.* A third outcome has been to substitute a less than helpful motor program for sound academic tutoring in such subjects as reading, while another less than helpful outcome has been to expose clumsy children to too narrow a range of motor activities (angles in the snow seems to be a favorite), a strategy which is not likely to elicit change in motor competencies. And finally, many children free of motor problems are placed in what are often stilted and overly structured programs of perceptual-motor training, children who if left free to play in normal ways would tax and thus improve their perceptual

---

* The day before this paper was written, I counseled a parent whose five-year-old boy, although posting a 126 in the verbal I.Q. of a recently administered intelligence test, was plagued with moderate neurological problems which made running impossible, and even standing and catching a ball tenuous. Having read some of the pronouncements mentioned above, the mother became concerned that her verbally intelligent, but motorically handicapped child would begin to evidence learning difficulties including the inability to read and the like!

and motor abilities to a far greater extent than occurs within the programs described.

What is also tragic is that within the research literature during the past twenty years are contained innumerable investigations which afford sound guidelines for what one may expect from various programs in which physical activity is an integral part. Moreover other literature illuminates the learning phenomena critical to determining whether engaging in movement changes anything (and if so, what).[5,7,8]

I have grown weary of talking and writing about research which illustrates quite clearly that movement experiences in which the child's mind is not involved will not change academic competencies. And thus I will not do so here.*

Rather it is my intent to explore three related issues which revolve around the question of what abilities will truly change when one inserts movement experiences in a program of education for children. These issues are labeled "transfer width," "intermediate variables" and intellectual mediation.

TRANSFER WIDTH. I believe I have chosen the most important issue to discuss first. It is critical, when evaluating outcomes of motor experiences for children, to determine just what *are* the relationships between program content and the objectives stated for that program. Relative to this type of inspection one is able to observe several possibilities. The first of these is a program in which little transfer-width is hypothesized, nor apparently hoped for, in which the content of the program exactly parallels the test used both at the beginning and the end. Some individuals employ the Frostig test and materials in this manner, while the Kephart Perceptual-Motor survey also lends itself to this type of "teaching-toward-the-test" practice.

On the other hand are individuals, some of whom use the same instruments listed above, who claim a variety of outcomes for programs in which the content consists of a few simple movement experiences. For the most part, these motor activities are not chosen or modified by the participating children, but are

---

* The interested reader may consult either the aforementioned *Physical Expressions of Intelligence* [1] or *Perceptual and Motor Development in Infants and Children.* [6]

rather arbitrarily administered by the all-knowing teacher-expert. It is this latter violation of logic and principles of learning which results in most cases of useless administration of movement experiences.

In contrast to this is the increasing awareness on the part of many educators that if one hopes to reach certain objectives in terms of measurable changes in exercise these behaviors must be inserted *in rather direct ways* into the content of the program. In diagram form both the illogical as well as the valid interpretation of the concept of transfer width is shown below.

Movement is a powerful tool, one which may be used to sharply hone a variety of abilities in children, if the activities are properly selected and administered. Our research, as well as other recent writings, outline not only how one may play a variety of reading games—activities to instill pre-reading competencies as well as all other academic abilities—but also how one may, in helpful, motivating and dramatic ways, encourage a child to engage in a variety of intellectual operations, ranging from memory work through evaluation to a number of types of problem solving. Moreover, it also seems possible to aid children to learn about human behavior, their own as well as that of others, if games and game situations are properly structured, planned and discussed.[3,4]

INTERMEDIATE VARIABLES. Programs of movement education often change other attributes for reasons not always apparent to the patient, and often warn the teacher. Indeed a teacher in a classroom is not always able to determine just *what* changed a child in her charge, after exposing him to not only her personality, but her concern, as well as to the content of the lessons.

Within an experimental setting it is important to factor out, and at times to cancel out, such things as tender-loving-care, special attention, and the positive changes these human attributes extended by the teacher might elicit. At the same time in the real world these efforts in human understanding *do* change childrens' self-concept which in turn motivates them to try harder in anything confronting them. James Oliver,[11] upon seeing changes of up to 25 per cent in the I.Q. scores of the retardates he exposed to a well-planned but totally physical education pro-

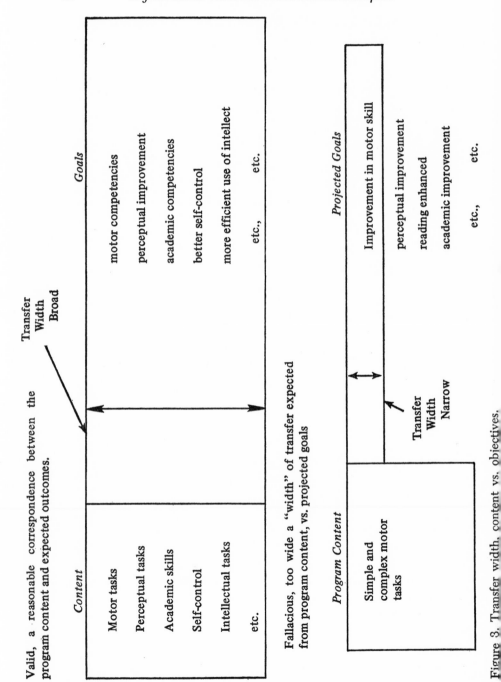

Figure 3. Transfer width, content *vs.* objectives.

gram, correctly assumed that the intermediate variable, the child's feelings about himself, had been modified, and in turn changed the effort each extended toward the second post-program administration of the intelligence test he used.

This dynamic theory of change may be diagrammed as follows and should be exploited whenever possible.

MOTIVATION, SELF-CONCEPT AS AN INTERVENING VARIABLE
IN A PROGRAM OF PERCEPTUAL-MOTOR EDUCATION

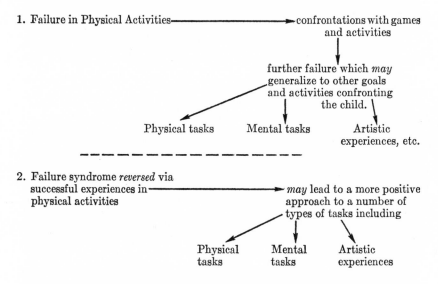

That is, children should be informed in very direct ways about how they have changed, how their performance has improved, and thus be led to perceive evidence which in turn will elicit more acceptable feelings about themselves. In programs we have assessed, we have found that physical performance measures are far easier to change than the child's feelings about himself or herself, particularly after only a five- to six-month interval. Thus one should not leave to chance the possibility that a child will feel better about himself because he can do more with his body. He must really believe it! Assessments of a teacher-educator are not enough. At the same time it is important not to rely *only* upon placebo effects of this nature. One should continually ask whether the *content* of the program is viable, and thus attempt to exclude the influences of the smile, energy, and good feelings of the benevolent teacher. These latter qualities are likely to make virtually anything work, particularly if the children dealt with have moderate motor, intellectual and/or emotional problems. Solid content, *plus* tender loving care, are both desirable elements of an effective program of physical activities.

Intellectual Mediation

It has been demonstrated in an ever increasing number of studies that if one desires to change intellectual abilities and/or academic proficiencies through movement experiences, opportunities for such activities should be built into the movement program. Moreover, as was pointed out above, if one desires to improve a child's self-concept, it is also desirable to involve the child in the "whys" of the program. That is, for best results in a program intended to improve movement abilities or other abilities, it is desirable not to treat the children involved like some kind of mechanical wind-up toys, but rather as advanced animals with the ability to think. Indeed some have said that the most outstanding intellectual feat of which humans are capable, and which indeed places them above animals in intelligence, is their ability to think about thought, to intellectualize about the intellect itself.

Thus if it is desired to aid a child to achieve self-control through various movement experiences (relaxation training, etc.), the participants should be given an exact awareness of just what the intent of the program is. Moreover if various types of memory tasks are presented to the child via movement experiences, again the youth should be informed just what is involved here, and to what it is hoped the movement activity will transfer. "You seem to have trouble remembering," the teacher might say. "These games may help you to remember your parent's instructions to you, the ways in which letters make up words, and the ways in which words make up sentences." The child should not have to grope for rationale underlying the experiences presented to him, but should be informed and be encouraged to think about the purpose of everything (to the limits of his understanding) to which he is exposed in programs of education, whether or not movement is an integral part.*

Summary

In summary it is believed that the following critical questions should be asked, and principles explored, when exposing children to programs in which movement plays a part. If the principles formulated and answers given are in line with current research it is unlikely that the theortical groundwork will be built upon sand, rather than upon a solid, scientific base. Points to consider are:

1. If one is going outside regular educational strategies, using movement activities to purportedly enhance such processes as reading, what transfer will occur which will bring back the movement program into the capacities really needed to read? †

2. If one wishes movement activities to enhance movement, the program should be preceded by a comprehensive program of evaluation and then activities chosen should not only pertain to the measured deficiencies, but should also be rather broad in nature, including a number of activities rather than a few.

3. For maximum transfer one should engage the mind of the learner in the reasons underlying all educational strategies whether or not they involve some kind of vigorous physical activity.

4. For maximum effectiveness, a program of perceptual-motor education should involve an environment and teaching atmosphere which is emotionally uplifting, *as well as* content which is carefully constituted relative to stated goals.

Movement is a powerful tool and for the most part constitutes a highly emotional experience in the life of children. Physical

---

* This same principle should be followed even if improved movement is the only goal, each drill should have a purpose and that purpose should be explained to athletes of all ages, for the drill to have the most lasting effect.[2]

† The processes needed to read well are numerous, and include word-shape to sound translation, reading with understanding, understanding the left-right principles, being able to place words in sentences properly, and the like. All of these *may* be taught via movement activities, but in truth are conceptual rather than physical in nature.[1,6]

experiences are thus seldom likely to have a neutral effect upon the mind and psyche of the maturing child. It behooves all of us to plan programs with scientifically sound objectives in mind and stated goals tied closely to laws of learning and principles of transfer. At the same time the quality of the motor activities we offer to children will be enhanced to the degree to which we involve children conceptually in decisions which must be made about any program in education.

BIBLIOGRAPHY

1. Cratty, B. J.: *Physical Expressions of Intelligence.* Englewood Cliffs, P-H, 1972.
2. ———, *Psychology in Contemporary Sport.* Englewood Cliffs, New Jersey: Prentice-Hall, 1973.
3. ———, *Intelligence in Action.* Englewood Cliffs, P-H, 1973.
4. ———, *Active Learning.* Englewood Cliffs, P-H, 1971.
5. ———, *Human Behavior: Exploring Educational Processes,* Wolfe City, University Pr, 1971, Ch. 8, Theoretical Approaches to Learning.
6. ———, *Perceptual and Motor Development in Infants and Children,* New York, Macmillan, 1970, Ch. 10, Evaluation and Discussion of Selected Perceptual-Motor Programs Purporting to Enhance Academic Functions.
7. ———. *Movement Behavior and Motor Learning,* 2nd ed. Philadelphia Lea & Febiger, 1967, Ch. 18, Transfer. (3rd. edition in press).
8. Ellis, Henry: *The Transfer of Learning.* New York, Macmillan, 1965.
9. Getman, G. N.: *How to Develop Your Child's Intelligence.* Luverne, Research Publication, 1952.
10. Kephart, Newell C.: *The Slow Learner in the Classroom.* Columbus, Merrill, 1960.
11. Oliver, James: The effects of physical conditioning exercises on the mental characteristics of educationally sub-normal boys. *Br J Educ Psychol, 28:*155–160, 1958.
12. Strauss, A. A. and Lehtinen, L. E.: *Psychopathology and the Education of the Brain Injured Child.* New York, Grune, 1947, vol. I, Fundamentals and Treatment.

USES OF MOVEMENT IN ELICITING "HIGH LEVEL" COGNITIVE ACTIVITY IN CHILDREN AND YOUTH*

I T IS APPARENT to many that the content of various programs of movement activities for children may be compared in several scales. For example, some are highly saturated with cognitive and/or academic elements, while others emphasize movements in reactions to highly structured instructions tendered by teachers. Some programs stress activities purportedly emphasizing perceptual development,[3] while others are obviously designed to enhance various academic and/or intellectual abilities.[4,11]

In general, the literature seems to indicate that the efficiency of a given program toward meeting its stated objectives is directly dependent upon the degree of congruence between the objectives and the content. It appears that many times the formulators of the various programs, in unrealistic ways, expect the content they recommend to transfer to too many or too wide a range of other abilities. Often the theoretical explanations that are offered, encourage those who practice these programs to expect too great a transfer width to emanate from the various activities suggested.

It is the purpose of the discussion which follows to suggest just what types of movement tasks appear to correspond to selected categories of intellectual functioning. The categories of

* Paper presented to the International Council of Sport and Physical Education sponsored by UNESCO, 11th Annual Meeting of the Research Committee, Rome, Italy, September 26 to October 1, 1971.

cognitive operations were arrived at by a survey of the literature, while the selection of motor activities was obtained from research carried out in the laboratory, as well as from surveying academic-motor and cognitive-motor programs.[6]

Although the matchings between motor activities and cognitive operations were arrived at without a great deal of empirical evidence, the following discussion may have several positive outcomes: (a) Some may be encouraged to determine, via research, whether the activities suggested may indeed serve to heighten the intellectual operations with which they have been paired; (b) others may take more care when making claims for intellectual development through movement experiences without careful consideration of program content; and (c) still others may, upon reviewing the information which follows, begin to expand programs of movement activities to include activities which encourage children to adopt a wider range of intellectual strategies than some of the program content presently appears to stimulate.

It has been decided to confine the discussion of intelligence to four primary categories. Initially, movement tasks which appear to enhance *memory* are grouped together. Next, various activities which may aid the individual to better *classify* various kinds of information are considered. The third category of intellectual functioning covered involves processes of *evaluation*. Within the final category have been placed various movement tasks which purportedly aid the child and youth to engage in *problem solving* behaviors.

MEMORY

Memorization has been listed by several scholars as one of the more basic intellectual operations.[2,10] Indeed, speculation about the many ramifications of human memory has a rich and interesting historical background. The ancient Greeks and Romans, for example, postulated and practiced various types of memory aids which are found in contemporary programs of self-improvement advertised commercially. The Greek orator, to facilitate his memory, often placed various parts of his speech within spatial reference points (i.e. rooms in the temple). Thus as he gave his speech he would "mentally travel" from room to room, upon whose walls he would imagine his works were inscribed.

IMITATION. It has been hypothesized by several writers that imitating the movements made by another individual may be a valid nonverbal test of body-image development, and thus may constitute a helpful way of enhancing the child's perceptions of his body, its parts, and its movement capacities.[1]

SHORT-TERM MEMORY SERIATION AND IMITATION. Several programs, including one already researched, contain tasks which purportedly enhance short-term memory via the imitation of movements presented in series. These programs may require a child to execute one or more of several operations.

1. Repeat in correct sequence a number of gestures, beginning with two, and then adding one at a time, after first visually inspecting the movements and then repeating them while blindfolded.[13]

2. Reproduce two or more body positions, with the demonstrator fixed, after visual inspection and reproduction also with vision.[13]

3. Reproduce a series of body positions originally presented via flash cards.[13]

4. Remembering and repeating a series of movements through a maze constructed of boxes or similar objects.[13]

5. Remember and repeat, in the same order, a series of bodily movements made within geometric configurations on the ground. Reproduction may be done via verbal directions or by first visually inspecting the series of movements and then repeating them.[4]

6. Remember and reproduce a series of locations to which a child has previously traveled.[4]

Several kinds of tasks are used in the various programs involving serial memory ability. McCormick,[13] for example, suggests that an ever-increasing series of movements may be made over a jump rope which is held or swings in various ways (i.e. overhead or back and forth in pendulum fashion).[13] A child may do something with a ball in two or more geometric configurations, to afford further interest.[4] At the same time, observational skills and descriptive language can be enhanced if a child who performs is not permitted to see the original demonstrator, but must rely upon the directions given verbally.[4]

LONG-TERM RETENTION OF SEMANTIC CONTENT. Long-term retention of semantic materials also has been studied by various researchers employing a movement approach. Spelling involves not only the retention of letter shapes but the rentention of letter series and word shapes. In previous research, it has been found that when using a phonics approach in learning letter shapes via movement, significant improvement is seen in children when contrasted to the scores achieved by children receiving extra tutoring but within an environment encouraging passivity rather than activity.[6,9]

CATEGORIZATION

Listed on most typologies of intellectual functioning are abilities which involve making discriminations; placing objects, events, symbols, etc., into categories; and similar classifying operations. The existence of this ability can be discerned in infants a few days old. Some have found that infants evidence the inclination to spend more time visually inspecting unfamiliar and/or unusual stimuli, than watching the familiar faces, shapes, and other events within close proximity.

As the infant matures, the ability to make increasingly complex discriminations, and to place objects, people, and events into increasingly discrete categories, are important criteria upon which to base assessments of intellectual functioning. By the time the child reaches school, he must not only discriminate between the various letter shapes in the alphabet, but must additionally recognize characteristics common to the 26 letters even though they may appear in different sizes, print styles, and locations within his space field. If his efforts at reading are to be successful, he must also categorize word shapes into innumerable categories representing a multitude of meanings.

Various programs of education in which movement plays a part have not contained a great many types of tasks which could conceivably enhance the child's ability to classify and to categorize. The tasks which have appeared in the various programs might themselves be placed within the following categories:

(a) Practice in pattern recognition constitutes the first category, in which various movement games and motor responses are encouraged with the use of large geometric figures placed on the playground. Thus, using these techniques, the attempt seems to be to aid children to place verbal labels on commonly seen geometric figures. These types of activities are designed to enhance the classification and categorization of what Guilford would term "figural content." [11]

(b) The letter recognition games, particularly if transfer is taught (for example, lower-case → upper-case → written letter → spoken letter → letter sound, etc.), represent another attempt through movement experiences to aid a child to form categories into which letters and letter combinations might be placed.

(c) In programs of movement education, a child may be asked to perform a movement within a given category, but at the same time may be permitted some latitude in his exact choice of movement. Thus, for example, an instructor may ask a child to "move down the mat a backwards way," or to "show me a hopping way to get into the hoop," etc.

(d) Various spatial concepts may be learned through movement experiences seen in several programs. A child may, for example, be asked to do something to the left or with the left (or right) side of his body, and in a similar manner may be asked to go under (or over) a chair or other obstacle to purportedly enhance acquisition of the spatial concepts of up-down and left-right. For instance, division of movements into four categories corresponding to up-down and left-right may be used.

The data emerging from the programs in which these activities have a part, is not extensive. However, in a study in which one of the objectives was to enhance children's verbal identification of geometric patterns (circle, square, half-circle, rectangle, and triangle), it was found that using a total-body movement approach was as successful as attempting to ingrain the same categorical concepts via small-group tutoring in a classroom environment. [6,9]

EVALUATION

Bloom places evaluative processes at the pinnacle of his taxonomy of the cognitive domain.[2] Similarly, his affective domain contains a level which he labels "characterization by a value or value complex." Guilford has also found a quality which he terms "sensitivity to problems," which he feels is closely related to an evaluative ability; moreover, his research has suggested that approximately eight different evaluative abilities exist, with the possibility of five more being uncovered as the result of further investigation.

Guilford suggests that evaluation involves the following sub-operations:

(a) comparing small differences, prior to classification of combinations of letters, numbers, etc.

(b) deciding whether there is logical consistency in verbal statements and/or visually presented scenes,

(c) detecting imperfections or irrelevancies within various contexts,

(d) deciding which of two or more kinds of information comes closer to satisfying a specific criterion.

More than one educator interested in enhancing cognitive processes has included exercises in evaluation in their workbooks and in automated programs for children and youth.[16] Several types of evaluative processes have been inserted into the programs of education, in which movement has also been inculcated. For example:

(a) An observing child may evaluate the quality of the movements made by another child or children, in response to such directions as "tell me if John performs his exercise well." [14]

(b) Quantitive aspects of movement experiences may also be evaluated by participation in programs of movement education: "How high did he jump?" "How many times did he do that?" "How fast did he run?"

(c) Self-evaluation may be encouraged in movement education programs. For example, to measure aspiration level and related measures, a child may be asked to estimate his future performance in a task prior to its execution. He may then be permitted to perform and subsequently be asked to make estimates of predicted successes on the third trial and those which follow.

It is difficult to locate definitive studies in which movement experiences have been demonstrated to enhance evaluative abilities. There are, in the literature, guidelines from several writers which should serve to direct the efforts of the more creative and flexible teachers, as well as focus the energies of diligent researchers.[4,14]

PROBLEM SOLVING

Another group of intellectual capacities may be termed "problem solving abilities." This category, similar to the previous ones discussed, is rather amorphous and is composed of several subabilities, depending upon which author one consults. This classification, however, is considered by most to be the highest level of intellectual functioning.

For example, the problem posed to a youngster may require him to *synthesize,* to put together information and/or movements in some meaningful and perhaps original manner. On the other hand, the problem may pose a dilemma which may be solved through *analysis,* the taking apart of a more complex problem and/or situation in order to extract meaning. Some complex problems require, to varying degrees, both processes of analysis and synthesis. For example, within a sports situation the player must analyze his own as well as his opponent's weaknesses and strengths; at the same time, he must consider how the synthesis of his teammates' abilities and shortcomings, paired with these same qualities in his opponent, may interact when they clash in an athletic contest.

Another continuum upon which problem solving behaviors may be studied, with reference to Guilford's work, is one at whose extremes may be placed the labels "convergent" and "divergent" thinking.[11] A problem may be structured so that there are a limited number of correct responses possible, or even only one appropriate decision called for. On the other hand, the intent may be to prompt the learner to explore and/or makeup a number of responses or conclusions. The former process would suggest *convergent* thought, one decision, while the latter suggests what is termed *divergent* thinking. It is unusual, however, to find that a problem solving situation calls for either an unlimited number of responses or is restricted to a single one. Therefore, one may construct a scale upon which may be placed a given kind of problem (movement problem or any other kind) relative to the degree of divergent or convergent thinking called for.

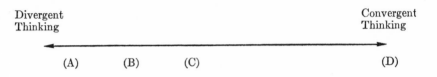

Divergent
Thinking

Convergent
Thinking

(A)   (B)   (C)   (D)

Examples of teacher-student interactions engaged in within programs of movement education, which might fall at several points within the continuum pictured, are as follows:

(A) Extreme divergent thinking would be expected to occur in response to the rather general directions "compose a dance routine."

(B) Less divergency would be expected if the directions "using movements of the trunk only," or "to be carried out within four minutes," or "taking place within a 10′ by 10′ square area," were to be added to the directions given in example "a" above.

(C) Moving toward the middle of the continuum, we might elicit reasonably focused, yet still somewhat unrestricted movement choices by suggesting that a child "find six ways of moving down the mat," or perhaps asking "how many ways can you start the 'trip' of a ball?". If the directions, "move six *backward* ways down the mat" were given, still more convergence of response is called for.

(D) Several extremely thoughtful problem solving situations have been described by writers which require the selection of a single movement solution. These lessons impose a number of conditions which, when met, permit the individual only a single response or responses within an extremely narrow band.

Piaget, in his writings, suggests several dimensions of problem solving behavior, usually not seen until adolescence, which are appropriate to consider for those dealing in movement as a learning modality.[18] These include:

A) POSSIBILITY-REALITY RELATIONSHIPS. Mature problem solving ability, according to Piaget, involves weighing what might be with what is. The mental manipulation of operations may only be handled in concrete terms earlier in the child's life.

B) COMBINATION PROPERTY. Piaget also emphasizes that mature thinking and logical operations seen in adolescents, may involve the putting together of hitherto unrelated aspects of the individual's reality. Others would call this quality "creative thinking," or perhaps the ability to synthesize information as previously described. In any case, if one accepts the validity of this quality, he should aid a child to obtain bits of the total he may need to solve a movement problem—perhaps parts of a sequence of movements needed to traverse a vertical or horizontal distance —and then permit the child to synthesize the pieces placed before him for consideration.

C) FLEXIBILITY. This quality of logical thought is emphasized in Piaget's writings as he discusses higher level thought processes. He suggests, for example, that as the youth becomes able to remove himself and his thoughts from concrete operations, he also becomes more flexible in seeking alternative solutions. This quality is similar to Guilford's various divergent thinking abilities discussed previously.

D) REVERSIBILITY. Increased mental capacity seen in older children and youth, Piaget suggests, also permits them to perceive the manner in which logical and concrete operations may be reversed. Examples of attempts to exploit this quality in programs of movement education might include seeking ways of both getting down as well as getting up a ladder, or perhaps seeking to move from one point to another, moving both forward and backward.

E) THEORIZING: DISCOVERING PRINCIPLES. Piaget,[17] as well as Gagné,[10] has suggested that the ability to discover a rule and to apply the rule of principle to more than one situation constitutes rather high level intellectual functioning. Mosston, in numerous examples, outlines how, within gymnastic lessons, basketball practices, and similar situations, students may be led toward the discovery of principles applicable to a wider range of situations than the one immediately encountered.

Mosston suggests the principle of "guided discovery," [14] a kind of Socratic approach in leading children toward the acquisition of principles which may underlie their physical performance. In this manner, it is suggested, the teacher already familiar with the final appropriate principle or principles, through judicious questioning and creating just the proper amount of cognitive dissonance in students, may aid the students to uncover principles and rules with reasonably broad applications.

SUMMARY, REVIEW

As there is relatively little data which ties, in direct ways, intellectual operations to specific kinds of movement experiences, much of the information contained in this discussion has been advanced in the form of unsupported hypotheses, rather than confirmed fact.

At the same time, deciphering relationships between the various intellectual levels reviewed, becomes difficult insofar as there is a considerable overlapping between functions various scholars have identified at the four levels dealt with. Certain subprocesses within the general ability level labeled "categorization," for example, are also found within the subdivision called "memorization." A similar overlap exists within various descriptions of *problem solving, creative thinking,* and other similar processes.

Further difficulty is encountered when attempting to synthesize behaviors as complex as the ones reviewed here, insofar as few authors and researchers agree upon similar classification systems. Different words are used to describe highly similar processes, or in other cases the same nomenclature is employed to describe processes which are dissimilar.

In any case, the available literature does indicate that if one has an objective to enhance various intellectual abilities through movement experiences, more than one cognitive operation should be built in to the tasks to which children and youth are exposed. The complexity and nature of the cognitive operations, which might be expected in youth of various ages, are illuminated in the writings of Piaget in particular.

Moreover, the writings of scholars interested in cognition and movement make it clear that the encouragement of youth to think in movement situations might be engendered (a) by gradually transferring decisions to the participating children, and (b) by taking into account the degree of diversity of response which is required when various instructions and situations are tendered to the participating youth.

Studies of intellectual ability indicate that this important category of human functioning is not an undifferentiated global whole, but rather is multifaceted.

Therefore, it appears that those constructing programs incorporating movement as a basic ingredient with the aim to elevate the participants' higher intellectual capacities, should take into account the diversity of the qualities they hope to modify.

BIBLIOGRAPHY

1. Berges, J. and Lezine I.: *The Imitation of Gestures.* London, The Spastics Society Medical Education and Information Unit in Association with William Heinemann Medical Books, 1965.
2. Bloom, Benjamin, (Ed.): *Taxonomy of Educational Objectives, Handbook I: Cognitive Domain.* New York, McKay, 1956.
3. Chaney, Clara and Kephart, Newell C.: *Motoric Aids to Perceptual Training.* Columbus, Merrill, 1968.
4. Cratty, B. J.: *Active Learning.* Englewood Cliffs, P-H, 1971.
5. ————: *Human Behavior and Learning: Understanding Educational Processes.* Wolfe City, University Pr, 1971.
6. Cratty, B. J. and Martin, Sister M. M.: *The Effects of a Program of Learning Games Upon Selected Academic Abilities in Children with Learning Difficulties.* Washington, D.C., Bureau of Health, Education and Welfare, Department of Education, Division of Handicapped Children, 1971.
7. Cratty, B. J.: *Physical Expressions of Intelligence.* Englewood Cliffs, P-H, 1971.
8. ————: Comparisons of verbal-motor performance and learning in serial memory tasks. *Res Q, 34:4,* December, 1963.
9. Cratty, B. J. and Szczepanik, Sister M.: *The Effects of a Program of*

Learning Games Upon Selected Academic Abilities in Children with Learning Difficulties, Part II. Washington, D.C., Bureau of Health, Education and Welfare, Department of Education, Division of Handicapped Children, 1971.

10. Gagné, R. W.: The analysis of instructional objectives for the design of instruction. In Glaser, Robert (Ed.): *Teaching Machines and Programmed Learning, II: Data and Directions*. Washington, D.C., Department of Audiovisual Instruction, National Education Association of the United States, 1965.

11. Guilford, J. P.: *Intelligence, Creativity, and their Educational Implications*. San Diego, Knapp, 1968.

12. Humphrey, James and Sullivan, Dorothy: *Teaching Slow Learners Through Active Games*. Springfield, Thomas, 1970.

13. McCormick, C., Schnobrich, J., and Footlik, S.: Willard, B. S., *Perceptual-Motor Training and Cognitive Achievement*. Downer's Grove, George Williams College, 1967.

14. Mosston, Muska: *Teaching Physical Education*. Columbus, Merrill, 1966.

15. Norman, D. A.: *Memory and Attention*. New York, Wiley, 1969.

16. Parnes, S. J.: *Student Workbook for Creative Problem-Solving Courses and Institutes*. Buffalo, New York: St U NY at Buffalo, 1961.

17. Piaget, J.: *The Language and Thought of the Child*. Translated by Gabain, M. London, Routledge and Kagan Paul, 1926.

18. ———; *The Origins of Intelligence in Children*. Translated by Cook, M. New York, Intl Univs Pr, 1952.

CHAPTER 5

READING PROCESSES AND
PERCEPTUAL-MOTOR ACTIVITIES*

D URING THE PAST TEN YEARS there have been an enormous number of writings dealing with the manner in which practice in various basic motor activities purportedly aid in the reading process. In previous writings, we have attempted to put to chase some of the more simplistic of these pronouncements.[7] In general, some of our critiques of theories relating movement behaviors to reading behaviors have been based upon several premises:

(a) Theortical arguments are only as valid as the data underlying the suppositions making up the theory.

(b) The act of reading consists of a number of complex subprocesses, which, if not smoothly functioning (either individually or in combination) are likely to be reflected in reading problems.

(c) Reading is largely an intellectual (cognitive) act, in which the problem is to translate a visual symbol to some kind of verbal-cognitive meaning.

There are types of movement activities, if properly employed, which may make a contribution to improving some of the subprocesses needed for some children to read well. It is the purpose of this outline to briefly illustrate the manner in which motor activities, carried out in specific ways, may contribute to better reading behavior on the part of some primary school children. The material which follows *will not*, it is hoped, be interpreted to mean that one should throw out some of the more traditional

---

* Prepared for a Symposium on Learning Disabilities, sponsored by The Manitoba Association for Learning Disabilities, held at the University of Manitoba, May, 1973.

ways of teaching reading, many of which have served children extremely well during the past decades. At the same time, reference to the materials contained in the following paragraphs, may encourage some teachers to approach some children in ways which are new and creative, and which thus may "break open" the child who is difficult to teach.

The processes which follow have been taken from a paper by John B. Carroll, Ph.D., which appears in a collection of reference papers from a Reading Forum sponsored by the National Institute of Neurological Diseases and Stroke, under the National Institutes of Health and the U.S. Department of Education. Other papers in this collection are excellent and should be reviewed by educators interested in various facets of teaching reading and learning to read.[*,3]

Carroll suggests that the following processes are usually agreed upon by most reading experts, although he also states that there is often controversy as to the *order* in which they should be acquired.

1. *The child must speak and understand the language with a reasonable skill level before he learns to read.* Piaget has suggested that language learning is accompanied in normal children by movement activities.[17,18] James Asher has devised a total program of language learning in which total bodily activities play a central role.[1]

2. *Children must learn to dissect spoken words into component sounds.* A number of phonics activities combined with vigorous motivating games have been employed for the past four years in the central city project which has been researched in the laboratory.[12] The Open Court method of phonics training was used for one year, for example.[10,11] Phonics games have also been devised by James Humphrey in his work at the University of Maryland.[14]

3. *The child must learn to recognize and discriminate the various letter forms to which he is exposed (lower case, upper case, manuscript, etc.).* In the central city program mentioned

---

* May be ordered from the Superintendent of Documents, U.S. Government Printing Office, Washington, D.C. 20402, for $2.00 (NINDS Monograph #11).

above, a considerable amount of effort has been expended to elicit the transfer referred to in number two. Games to facilitate upper to lower case translation have been devised, and the data indicated their success. Blackboards have been placed adjacent to mats and grids containing upper and lower case letters to facilitate this process.[4]

4. *The child must learn the left-right principle by which words are spelled and put into order in a continuous text.* This quality has been referred to by some perceptual-motor "magicians" as the "only" ability needed to read well. And conversely, if this trait is absent, it is further suggested, the reading process will be completely blocked. While the research does not support these pronouncements in their entirety, it is apparent that movement activities in which left-right directions and movements are emphasized, if properly transferred to left-right judgments in visual space, *may* enhance this left-right concept. However, concentrating only upon left-right games in which the body is moving will not, in itself, correct letter reversal. Additionally, research by several scholars indicates that left-right discrimination of body parts is not predictive of letter reversal problems in children.[2]

5. *The child must learn that various sounds are probable outcomes of various letter combinations, so that he may either recognize in print words that are commonly heard, or conversely, so that he can attempt to pronounce words seen for the first time.* The phonics games referred to previously under number two, are appropriate for instilling this quality in children.

6. The child must learn to recognize printed words by referring to a number of cues: their general shape, the letters composing them, the sounds the letters represent, as well as the meanings suggested by their context. A number of reading games have been devised, by Humphrey as well as by Cratty and his colleagues, which have been found, through research, to aid in sight recognition of words.[10,11,14]

7. *The child must be able to translate spoken words and phrases to written words and phrases, and vice versa.* A number of coding experiences may be employed, in which movement is

an integral part. These have been outlined in a text by Cratty. Additionally, some of the games contained in the text by Sullivan and Humphrey give children this kind of coding practice.[9,14]

8. *The child must learn to reason and to think about what is read, to the limits of his capacity and talent.* Following directions, reading comprehension and other related qualities are contained in a number of texts [6,9] in the bibliography of this chapter. Games in which children are encouraged to engage in a variety of cognitive processes and to verbalize their speculations and solutions to various problems are helpful within this context.

There are numerous valid strategies and methods which have been found effective in the teaching of reading and in the remediation of reading problems, most of which exclude a great deal of movement on the part of the child. The methods referred to on the previous pages, however, contain strategies in which the child is most of the time encouraged to move in various ways. This type of approach has been found to be helpful to some of the children for at least three reasons:

(a) The activities are motivating and fun.
(b) They encourage close undivided attention on the part of the child participating.
(c) They match the obvious movement needs of some children, with curriculum content compatible to these needs.

Movement activities are potentially powerful tools in educational programs for both normal and atypical children. Their effective use depends upon the selection of correct program content, compatible with projected goals.

BIBLIOGRAPHY

1. Asher, James J.: The total physical response approach to second language learning. *Mod Language J*, vol. LIII, no. 1, January, 1969.
2. Ayres, Jean A.: Patterns of perceptual-motor dysfunction in children: A factor analytic study. *Percept Mot Skills*, Monograph Suppl., I–V20, 1965.
3. Carroll, John B.: The nature of the reading process. In *Reading Forum:* NINDS Monograph No. 11, Calkins, Eloise O., Ed. Bethesda, National Institute of Neurological Diseases and Stroke, Public Health

Service, National Institutes of Health, U.S. Department of Health, Education, and Welfare, 1969.
4. Cratty, Bryant J.: *Active Learning.* Englewood Cliffs, P-H, 1971.
5. ———: Evaluation and discussion of selected perceptual-motor programs purposting to enhance academic function. In *Perceptual and Motor Development in Infants and Children.* New York, Macmillan, 1970.
6. ———: *Learning and Playing: Fifty Vigorous Activities for the Atypical Child.* Freeport, Educational Activities, 1968.
7. ———: *Physical Expressions of Intelligence.* Englewood Cliffs, P-H, 1972.
8. ———: *Human Behavior: Exploring Educational Processes.* Wolfe City, University Pr, 1971.
9. Cratty, Bryant J. and Szczepanik, Sister Mark: *Sounds, Words, and Actions.* Freeport, Educational Activities, 1971.
10. ———: *The Effects of a Program of Learning Games Upon Selected Academic Abilities of Children with Learning Difficulties.* Washington, D.C., Bureau of Education for the Handicapped, U.S. Office of Education, 1970.
11. Cratty, Bryant J. and Martin, Sister Margaret Mary: *The Effects of a Program of Learning Games Upon Selected Academic Abilities of Children with Learning Difficulties.* Washington, D.C., Bureau of Education for the Handicapped, U.S. Office of Education, 1970.
12. Cratty, Bryant J., Ikeda, Namiko, Martin, Sister Margaret Mary, Jennett, Clair, and Morris, Margaret: *Movement Activities, Motor Ability and the Education of Children.* Springfield, Thomas, 1970.
13. Frostig, Marianne and Maslow, Phyllis: *Movement Education: Theory and Practice.* Chicago, Follett, 1970.
14. Humphrey, James H. and Sullivan, Dorothy D.: *Teaching Slow Learners Through Active Games.* Springfield, Thomas, 1970.
15. Myers, Patricia I. and Hammill, Donald, D.: *Methods for Learning Disorders.* New York, Wiley, 1969.
16. Piaget, Jean: *The Language and Thought of the Child.* Translated by Gabain, M. London, Routledge & Kagan Paul, 1926.
17. ———: *The Origins of Intelligence in Children.* Translated by Cook, M. New York, Intl Univs Pr, 1952.
18. Wedemeyer, Avaril and Cejka, Joyce: *Learning Games for Exceptional Children: Arithmetic and Language Development Activities.* Denver, Love Publishing Company, 1971.

PART II

MOVEMENT ABILITIES IN EARLY CHILDHOOD: THEORY AND GUIDELINES

CHAPTER 6

SOME MEANINGS OF MOVEMENT IN EARLY CHILDHOOD*

Introduction

A NUMBER OF BASIC QUESTIONS usually arise among a group of preschool and elementary school educators concerned with the roles of physical activity, physical education, movement, and/or some kind of perceptual-motor training within the school environment. Basically, these queries revolve around who should have what kinds of activities, and the worth of various programs of structured or unstructured motor activity upon various facets of the child's personality. It is with some of these questions that the material on the following pages attempts to deal.

Why Programs of Movement in the Schools?

Various philosophical commitments to the role of movement activities within the educational context, discernable upon a perusal of history, still prevail within modern schools and school systems. Some teachers feel uncomfortable with noisy, active children, despite the fact that their noise and activity may be directed toward desirable educational ends. Others require quiet, conforming passivity at all times ("No talking on the lunch benches!") while still others believe that there are certain times when the bodies of children should be permitted to move (i.e. at recess), while at other times these same children should be outwardly passive, while inwardly their young minds should be permitted and indeed encouraged to churn.

---

* Prepared for the National Leadership Institute in Early Childhood Development in Washington, D.C., October 14 and 15th, 1971.

The research supports the suggestion that even from birth children seem to have basic individual differences in their needs for and propensities to move. In one study, for example, some babies evaluated shortly after birth were seen to be about 150 times more active than the more passive infants.[14,22] Other investigations document the often-observed fact that nursery school children display marked individual differences in the amount of vigor which each brings to the play yard, differences which persist into adulthood.[15]

By the time youngsters enter the first grade, many of them are beginning to form reasonably exact opinions concerning their own movement capacities, and how these compare to the abilities of others in their play groups. There are probably at least two main reasons for lack of participation in playground games on the part of a child entering elementary school: (a) perceived lack of ability and competency, and/or (b) some kind of emotional problem which reflects a disinclination to participate.

In general, the research supports the institution of sound programs of movement experiences for preschool and elementary school children for the reasons listed below:

(a) Physical competencies developed in play and in more structured physical education periods will add to a child's general feelings of competency.[7]

(b) Creative movement skills encouraged through various forms of artistic expression, and in movement games in which choice behavior is encouraged in children, are likely to result in more qualitative participation in all forms of social interaction taking place within the elementary school.[9]

(c) Active children, if confined too long, will likely bring less enthusiasm to classroom tasks confronting them. For example, in one study carried out in Scandinavia, a group of fit children, following four hours of test taking and study, performed less capably in a final Intelligence Quotient test than did less fit children, despite the fact that the two groups performed equally well in a similar I.Q. test at the beginning of the day. The investigators suggested that prolonged confinement of children who are fit and thus probably have high activity needs, may be contraindicated in elementary schools.[18]

(d) Movement in children is seemingly an inherent need which, if stifled, will often lead to less desirable behaviors. This same "play-need" in animals, has been well documented in the literature.

(e) Vigorous activities practiced with high levels of motivation on the part of children, will result in greater levels of muscular and cardiovascular fitness.

MOVEMENT AND INTELLIGENCE

While the majority of the correlative studies have demonstrated, however, that the stereotype of the bright but unfit elementary school child is not very accurate, in groups of children with learning problems it will usually be found that there is a greater percentage with coordination and fitness problems than would be found in a group of so-called normal children.[7] However, most of the time, when any desirable traits of children are measured—whether they be social competency, intelligence, muscular fitness, or some similar quality—they show a slight positive correlation with each other.

At the same time, when a normal child reaches two years of age, one group of researchers has identified two separate families of attributes in children. In one group were test scores evaluating tasks whose performance depended primarily upon motor competency. A second domain contained scores which, even at age two reflected intellectual ability.[16]

It is thus to be expected that early measures of competency, primarily motor in nature, are poor predictors of later intelligence. In one longitudinal study, for example, it was found that the silent, contemplative, relatively passive male infants were more intelligent in their later years than were the more active ones.[10]

Many of the studies which have attempted to positively change I.Q. scores through movement have employed retarded children as subjects. Although the earliest of these found that a good physical education program seemed to cause I.Q. scores to ascend (25% in one case), these scholars attributed the change to an improvement in self-concept.[17]

The findings from more recent studies, employing adequate controls, suggest that while fitness measures improve, more global measures of personality and intelligence do not necessarily show a parallel rise when retarded children are exposed to traditional physical education activities.

However, two investigations, carried out in the past few years, offer helpful guidelines when attempting to improve a child's intellectual functioning by the application of movement programs. In both these studies, positive findings were obtained when children were given movement problems to work out, in small groups or individually (e.g. "see how many ways you can find to jump over the line"). When these kinds of motor tasks are paired with various thought problems, a child's ability to think more efficiently has a better chance of being improved.[20,24]

Academic Operations and Motor Activity

During the past twenty years, a number of books as well as numerous articles in the popular press, have described programs containing motor activities which purportedly improve various academic operations. It is often suggested that reading, spelling, and similar tasks will be enhanced if teachers will only engage in various kinds of perceptual-motor, sensory-motor, or some similarly named experiences.*

However, the available research literature on this general topic, suggests that many of these pronouncements should be weighed carefully before a teacher proceeds out of the normal channels usually employed to teach academic skills in the elementary school program. The teacher should ask herself (or himself) whether various movement experiences will indeed be more efficient in promoting hopeful academic outcome, than would continued use of traditional methods of teaching reading, spelling, various prereading concepts, and mathematical skills.

Indeed, the data should urge all but the most indoctrinated individuals to exercise extreme caution when employing some type of movement panacea to rectify an academic operation.

---

* A documented review of the validity of these theories, and the results of current research findings which they seem to have inspired is found in reference 9 in the bibliography.

Many of the movement experiences advocated are far removed in a developmental standpoint from the academic operations to which they will purportedly transfer.

A large number of studies utilizing elementary children with and without reading problems, have also revealed that the likelihood of improving reading via some kind of exposure to movement tasks, is remote indeed.[9] Some of the findings suggest that not only will academic operations be unaffected, but that some of the so-called perceptual-motor abilities inherent in the training program will similarly not be improved.[12]

It *is* found however that when various academic operations are incorporated *directly* into various movement games, these operations are likely to be improved upon. In several studies, more improvement was forthcoming in such traditional classroom skills as letter recognition, reading, spelling, pattern recognition, and similar operations using various movement games than was evident when control groups in these same investigations were exposed to traditional small-group tutoring within a more passive classroom environment.[6,7,10]

CHILDREN WITH MOVEMENT PROBLEMS

The best estimates emanating from investigations of elementary school children, suggest that 15 to 18 per cent of a population of normal children (from which the obviously impaired have been culled out) evidence various movement problems which can be attributed to some kind of structural impairment in the nervous system.[19] These thousands of children with minimal to moderate neurological impairments, enter elementary schools all over the country each year, and attempt to function and compete in various kinds of motor tasks with the average to superior child, and invariably lose.

These children may be expected to evidence not only an inability to play well at recess and during physical education, but also cannot efficiently translate their thoughts, via handwriting, to paper within the regular school day. Studies we have carried out at the University of California at Los Angeles indicate that such children suffer from marked problems involving their self-concept, far more than do ordinary children. Their friends make fun of them, boys and girls do not like them, and in other ways they do not measure up socially to the expectations of their peers.[7]

This group of clumsy children often is either too under-aroused or overaroused, and too active to learn well in the ordinary classroom. Usually these children have significantly lower performance I.Q.'s (based upon the execution of perceptual-motor tasks including drawing geometric figures), than verbal I.Q.'s.

Evaluation of Motor Difficulties

It would appear that it is contingent for the teacher to attempt to survey her class within the first days of each school year in an effort to identify the children with possible movement problems. She should sample each child's ability to engage in fine manipulative activity and writing tasks, as well as his competency in controlling his larger muscle groups and integrating them in meaningful tasks.

Various measures of self-control may also be utilized by teachers. Studies have shown that such measures obtained when children are asked to move as slowly as they can in various tasks, are predictive of general self-control in classrooms as well as of potential success in various academic tasks. In a recent unpublished study, for example, children at the first grade level were asked to walk a line twelve feet long placed on the floor, as "slowly as you can." First grade children who complete this type of task in much under fifteen seconds, may be the same children who have difficulty sitting still in the classroom and attending to their work for the prolonged periods of time required of them by first grade teachers. The correlation between measures of this nature and academic performance are reasonably high in several studies which have been carried out since 1965.

It is usually found that some type of balance measure is most predictive of scores in a wide range of tasks requiring large muscle control. First-grade children, for example, should be able to stand, without falling over or walking, in a reasonably immobile position with their feet close together and parallel to each other.

Various tasks involving manipulative ability might be employed to evaluate manual dexterity. Finger opposition is a helpful assessment task, in which a child is asked to touch, in quick order, the fingers of one hand to the thumb of the same hand.

A child at the first grade level should be able to draw a reasonably accurate circle and square, and should copy both a square and rectangle so that their differences are apparent. By the time a child is seven, he should be able to draw a reasonably accurate triangle, and by eight, a diamond. As a child enters the first grade, he should be able to block print in letters about two inches high, his first (but not his last) name. His ability to print letters, of course, increases with age while the size of the letters he can manage decreases.

By the age of seven, most children can skip, and (75% of the time) can identify their left and right hands, feet, and other body parts. Girls and boys at seven, can quickly oppose each finger of one hand to the thumb of the same hand. Children at this age can also hop with accuracy into small squares about 1' by 1' in size.[9]

By the age of eight, most children can transfer a hopping pattern rhythmically from one foot to the other, i.e. two hops on one foot and then two on the other. Eight-year-olds can jump, both feet together, over a stick about twelve inches high, and can broadjump from a standing position, slightly over three feet.

It also seems important to emphasize what five-year-olds *cannot* usually accomplish, for frequently one encounters false norms for this age group. A five-year-old cannot, without special training, be expected to consistently identify correctly his left and right body parts better than what would be expected by chance. A five-year-old cannot hop rhythmically from one foot to the other in either a two-hops-two-hops pattern, in a three-hops-three-hops pattern, or in a more difficult pattern (i.e. two hops, to three hops on the other foot). Similarly, most five-year-olds cannot balance in an immobile, controlled manner with one foot ahead of the other, in a heel-to-toe position. To expose five-year-olds to these tasks and then assign the failures to some type of structured, perceptual-motor training program will usually result in most of a kindergarten population being so designated.

Research does indicate that the performance scores of many children with coordination problems can be changed due to training.[7] Whether the nature of this change is due to the fact that such children learn to circumvent their problems by adopting new strategies when performing motor skills, or whether some kind of subtle neurological modifications take place within their nervous systems, is not known, and perhaps not highly important. What is important is that with patient, motivating, and nonstressful help, they can be improved.

Remediation

In general, research has indicated that the most marked changes can be elicited in measures of strength and fitness over the shortest period of time. The strength and endurance of children can be improved within a few weeks, if exercises are applied at the end of training periods held two or three times weekly, for brief periods of time.

Next in order of expected improvement are qualities involving various movements denoting the accuracy of bodily adjustments. Activities in which the arms and legs must be integrated in some way, such as jumping and throwing movements and various balance activities, are also employer. The guidelines suggested by the literature for the improvement of these qualities, are as follows:

(a) A variety of activities should be utilized. Several kinds of balance tasks should be employed, for example: those in which the body is held static in some manner, i.e. a one foot balance, and others in which the child is asked to traverse a line on the floor or to walk a balance beam.

(b) Agility of several types should be incorporated into a program for a child evidencing the inability to move his body well. Activities may involve various kinds of locomotor tasks; hopping, jumping, skipping, etc., as well as those similar to various, simple tumbling movements; rolling like a log, front and back shoulder rolls of various types * and various ways of get-

---

* Caution should be exercised when persuading young children to execute the traditional back and front rolls, for if their arm strength is insufficient, rather severe neck strains can occur.

ting up and down from the floor to a standing position and back.

(c) Ball throwing and catching tasks should be offered the child sequentially, from the easier ones to the more difficult. For example, a child who has trouble catching a ball thrown on the fly, may become more successful by sitting and intercepting a larger ball rolled to him on the floor. A child having trouble batting a ball when thrown to him, may be helped by hitting an immobile, volleyball-size missile, teed up in front of him on a traditional batting T.

(d) As children grow older and/or more competent, the percentages of the more basic activities, i.e. balance, agility, and the like, may be diminished in their improvement program and the percentage of specific sports skills enlarged. Younger children, or those with more pronounced movement problems, should be kept longer on the more basic activities involving simple bodily integrations. The more successful children, and those who are older (and from whom the culture demands specific competencies) should be exposed to the exact skills needed in traditional games. Batting balls, throwing, and the like should be introduced into their program as these same skills begin to appear in the games their peers are playing.

(e) In general, a training period involving gross motor activity should be from thirty minutes to an hour in length, and offered from two to five times a week. The period may begin with basic agility and balance movements, and continue with the introduction of sports skills and the opportunity to work at simple games. The period should terminate with exercises and various activities intended to relax the child and to reduce his activation to the level necessary for him to successfully participate in the classroom to which he may be returning.

(f) Remediation of fine motor skills including handwriting and printing, may also be given on a daily basis form twenty to thirty minutes, which research indicates is optimum. Children who cannot accurately execute various letters in printed form, may be provided with shallow pans of modeling clay in which writing implements may be used. This offers greater stability and accuracy, and also slows down their movements, perhaps offering them a better opportunity to visually track their moving stylus.

(g) There is a reasonable amount of persuasive evidence available to indicate that significant changes in motor ability measures, including balance and agility as well as printing and writing performance, may be elicited from hyperactive, incoordinate children placed on the proper kinds and dosages of medication.

(h) Research also indicates that the clumsy child not given some kind of success in motor activities, is likely to regress by the time he reaches late childhood or early adolescence. At the same time, there is further evidence to indicate that if a motor education program is discontinued for a period of time (in one study for 3 months), the physically inept child is also likely to regress.

Activating and Calming

There is a good deal of evidence indicating that vigorous physical activities arouse children physiologically and psychologically. There are a number of interesting findings which outline several types of relationships between academic learning and activating and calming activities.

Research in Czechoslovakia as well as in this country, in recent years, has indicated that carefully planned programs of various kinds of relaxation and impulse-control training can help some children to evidence better self-control, an improvement which is often accompanied by better classroom learning.[2,6,10] This kind of training is often useful immediately following vigorous physical activities, but may be applied to some children, whenever they need it during the school day. Preliminary studies attest to the potential worth of this type of activity for children who are hard to manage, or who have a difficult time managing themselves.

SUMMARY AND OVERVIEW

The available research outlines several guidelines through which motor activities may be integrated more effectively into the preschool and primary school program. Consideration of these guidelines and the practices they in turn suggest, should help teachers deal more effectively with the normal child, with the boy or girl evidencing learning problems, and with the atypical child.

1. Indices of motor ability correlate very slightly with measures of intelligence. However, the correlations are higher within groups of children less capable intellectually, or when the motor tasks contrasted to the I.Q. measures are highly complex.

2. Studies that were well controlled, in which I.Q. measures have changed in both normal and mildly retarded children due to exposure to traditional physical education and fitness programs, have usually elicited the observation from the researcher involved, that the improvement was due to a heightening of the child's self-concept through increased proficiency in game participation.[17]

3. Academic operations have been demonstrated to be improvable through movement experiences, only when the operations (i.e. spelling, letter recognition, reading, etc.) are combined in *direct ways* with the games and movements presented to the children.[6,10]

4. It has been demonstrated that clumsy boys of ten, performing poorly in physical skills possess a low self-concept, and often prefer to play games inappropriate to members of their sex.[7]

5. There are reasonably precise indices of large as well as fine motor functioning through which a preschool or primary school teacher may survey her class during their first days together each year. These measures should include those tasks evaluating writing behavior, manipulative abilities, large muscle control as well self-control.

6. Remediation of minor motor problems, particularly in younger children, does seem possible upon consulting the available literature, if regular periods two to five times weekly are devoted to developmental activities of a comprehensive nature directly related to the nature of each child's problems.[7]

7. Methods of deactivating and activating children so that they perform at an optimum in both classroom tasks and in playground activities, have been shown to be effective. These techniques may be applied to activate habitually sleepy children, or

to calm children whose arousal and activity levels are, most of the time, inappropriate for good concentration upon their work in the classroom.[2,7]

NEEDED RESEARCH

A great deal of research is needed in order to formulate more accurate guidelines than were presented on these pages. For example:

1. Longitudinal studies are needed to accurately describe the possible influence of preschool education in which motor activities may play a central role upon the later academic performance and personal adjustment of children entering elementary school.

2. Further explorations are needed of various sex differences as they may effect the many possible interactions between motor capacities, movement needs and academic performance.

3. More valid norms are needed through which to more accurately evaluate the motor abilities of elementary school and pre-elementary school boys and girls. Such norms should reflect not only sex differences, but possible racial and ethnic differences in these traits.

BIBLIOGRAPHY

1. Bayley, Nancy: Behavioral correlates of mental growth—birth to thirty-six years. *Am Psychol, 23*:117, January, 1968.
2. Bednarova, V.: An investigation concerning the influence of psychotonic exercise upon the indices of concentration of attentiveness. *Teor Prax Teles Vychov, 16*:437–442, 1968.
3. Bloom, Benjamin: *Stability and Change in Human Characteristics.* New York, Wiley, 1964.
4. Bower, T. G.: The visual world of infants. *Sci Am, 215*:80–97, 1966.
5. Cawley, John F., Goodstein, Henry, and Burrow, Will: *Reading and Psychomotor Disability Among Mentally Retarded and Average Children.* Storrs, School of Education, U of Conn, 1968.
6. Cratty, Bryant J. and Martin, Sister Margaret Mary: *The Effects of a Program of Learning Games upon Selected Academic Abilities in Children with Learning Difficulties, Part I.* Washington, D.C., U.S. Office of Education, Bureau of Handicapped Children, 1970.
7. Cratty, Bryant J., Ikeda, Namiko, Martin, Sister Margaret Mary, Jennett, Clair, and Morris, Margaret: *Movement Activities, Motor*

Ability and the Education of Children. Springfield, Thomas, 1970.

8. Cratty, Bryant J.: *Active Learning.* Englewood Cliffs, P-H, 1971.

9. Cratty, Bryant J.: *Perceptual and Motor Development in Infants and Children.* New York, Macmillan, 1970.

10. Cratty, Bryant J. and Szczepanik, Sister Mark: *The Effects of a Program of Learning Games upon Selected Academic Abilities in Children with Learning Difficulties, Part II.* Washington D.C., U.S. Office of Education, Bureau of Handicapped Children, 1971.

11. Cratty, Bryant J. and Szczepanik, Sister Mark: *Sounds, Words, and Actions.* Freeport, Long Island, New York: Educational Activities, 1971.

12. Fisher, Kirk L.: *Effects of a Structured Program of Perceptual-Motor Training on the Development and School Achievement of Educable Mentally Retarded Children,* Washington, D.C., U.S. Office of Health, Education and Welfare, Office of Education, Bureau of Research, 1969.

13. Humphrey, James and Sullivan, Dorothy: *Teaching Slow Learners Through Active Games.* Springfield, Thomas, 1970.

14. Irwin, Q. C.: Amount of mobility of 73 newborn infants. *J Comp Psychol, 14:*415, 1932.

15. Kagan, J. and Moss, H. A.: *Birth to Maturity: A Study in Psychological Development.* New York, Wiley, 1962.

16. Meyers, C. E. and Dingman, Harvey F.: Structure of abilities at the preschool ages: Hypothesized domains. *Psychol Bull, 57:*514–32; 1960.

17. Oliver, James: The effects of physical conditioning exercises and activities on the mental characteristics of educationally sub-normal boys. *Br J Educ Psychol, 28:*155, 1958.

18. Railo, Willi S.: Physical and mental endurance, and Physical fitness and intellectual achievement, Unpublished report. Oslo, Norwegian College of Physical Education and Sport, 1968.

19. Rappaport, Sheldon: *Public Education for Children with Brain Dysfunction.* Syracuse, Syracuse U Pr, 1969.

20. Rarick, Lawrence, and Broadhead, Geoffrey: *The Effects of Individualized Versus Group Oriented Physical Education Programs on Selected Parameters of the Development of Educable Mentally Retarded and Minimally Brain Injured Children.* Sponsored by the United States Office of Education and the Joseph P. Kennedy, Jr. Foundation, 1968.

21. Rutherford, William L: Perceptual-motor training and readiness. *Reading and Inquiry,* Figurel, J. Allen (Ed.). International Reading Association, Conference Proceedings, X, 194–196, 1965.

22. Scarr, Sandra: Genetic factors in activity motivation. *Child Dev, 37:*663–73, 1966.

23. Smith, O. W., and Smith, P. C.: Developmental studies of spatial judg-

ments by children and adults. *Percept Mot Skills,* monograph supplement, 22:3–73, no. 1, 1966.

24. Widdop, J. H., Barton, P., Cleary, B., Proyer, V. A. and Wall, A. E.: *The Effects of Two Programmes of Physical Education Upon the Behavioral and Psychological Traits of Trainable Retarded Children,* a study financed by the Quebec Institute of Research in Education, contract no. 68–AS–11–04–02. Montreal, McGill University, 1969.

PERCEPTUAL-MOTOR BEHAVIORS
CHECK LIST

THE FOLLOWING TASKS are reasonable to expect in 75 to 80 per cent of the children of the indicated ages. Children should be tested individually.

The data upon which this is based has been collected from children in white middle-class neighborhoods.

A child failing to master four to six of the tasks for his or her age probably needs (a) a more thorough evaluation and (b) some kind of remedial help.

Various sex differences are indicated.

Two to Three Years

	YES	NO
1. Displays a variety of scribbling behavior.	____	____
2. Can walk rhythmically at an even pace.	____	____
3. Can step off low object, one foot ahead of the other.	____	____
4. Can name hands, feet, head, and some face parts.	____	____
5. Opposes thumb to fingers when grasping objects and releases objects smoothly from finger-thumb grasp.	____	____
6. Can walk a two-inch wide line placed on ground, for ten feet.	____	____

Four to Four and a Half

	YES	NO
1. Forward broadjump, both feet together and clear of ground at the same time.	——	——
2. Can hop two or three times on one foot without precision or rhythm.	——	——
3. Walks and runs with arm action coordinated with leg action.	——	——
4. Can walk a circular line a short distance.	——	——
5. Can draw a crude circle.	——	——
6. Can imitate a simple line cross using a vertical and horizontal line.	——	——

Five to Five and a Half

	YES	NO
1. Runs thirty yards in just over eight seconds or less.	——	——
2. Balances on one foot (girls 6–8 seconds) (boys 4–6 seconds).	——	——
3. Child catches large playground ball bounced to him chest-high from fifteen feet away; four to five times out of five.	——	——
4. Rectangle and square drawn differently (one side at a time).	——	——
5. Can hi-jump eight inches or higher over bar with simultaneous two-foot take off.	——	——
6. Bounces playground ball, using one or two hands, a distance of three to four feet.	——	——

Six to Six and a Half

	YES	NO
1. Can block print first name in letters 1½ to 2 inches high.	——	——
2. Can gallop, if it is demonstrated.	——	——
3. Can exert six pounds or more of pressure in grip strength measure.	——	——

4. Can walk balance beam 2 inches wide, 6 inches high, and 10 to 12 inches long. ——— ———
5. Can run sixty feet in about five seconds. ——— ———
6. Can arise from ground from back lying position, when asked to do so as fast as he can, in two seconds or under. ——— ———

Seven to Seven and a Half

                                                    YES   NO

1. Left hand and other left-right body parts identified. ——— ———
2. Can draw triangle. ——— ———
3. Can do standing broadjump of 35 inches or more, or can execute vertical jump of 6 inches more than total standing height plus reach with arm extended upward. ——— ———
4. Girls can do jumping jacks in rhythm. Boys can posture ten seconds on one foot, keeping other foot in place. ——— ———
5. Can quickly and accurately oppose each finger of one hand to the thumb of the same hand (girls). Can do finger opposition as described above, but with the need to visually inspect movements (boys). ——— ———
6. Can jump and hop accurately into squares one foot by one foot in size. ——— ———

Eight to Eight and a Half

                                                    YES   NO

1. Can skip or hop rhythmically, twice on one foot and then twice on other, several cycles. ——— ———
2. Can draw diamond when shown model. ——— ———
3. Can do standing broadjump forty inches or more or can high jump, two feet take off simultaneously, over twelve inches or more in height. ——— ———

4. Can throw small ball thirty feet or more.   ———   ———
5. Can run thirty yards in 6.5 seconds or faster (less).   ———   ———
6. Boys can execute rhythmic jumping jack movement and can demonstrate quick opposition of fingers to thumb, in five seconds or less (first finger to thumb, and back again, of one hand).   ———   ———

CHAPTER 8

MATURATION AND CHANGE IN ABILITY TRAITS: IMPLICATIONS FOR EDUCATORS*

THE FOLLOWING OUTLINE is taken from material in two texts [3,4] containing a model which attempts to depict the manner in which the human abilities tend to diffuse, and become integrated as maturation takes place.

Essentially the model rests upon the following principles and assumptions:

1. Rudimentary evidence of abilities within four categories may be seen in infants near birth. These include the beginnings of intellectual, perceptual, motor, and verbal behavior.

2. As the infant matures the number of separate abilities within each of the four channels proliferates, and diffuses.

3. The rate of diffusion of abilities, and the appearance of various, discrete abilities within the various channels may be triggered either by inherent automatic mechanisms, or by exposure of the child to various environmental conditions.

4. Due to either inherent defects or environmental circumstances, the diffusion of abilities within a given channel (verbal, cognitive, motor, and perceptual) may to varying degrees be blunted. That is, a given child may for various reasons evidence an unevenness in his development, moving ahead in a normal way intellectually, for example, while giving evidence of motor problems; or perhaps proceeding well verbally while evidencing perceptual deficits.

---

* Prepared for the Conference in Learning Disabilities, Little Rock, Arkansas, April, 1973.

5. As maturation continues, the child will build bonds between various abilities within the same developmental channel, or between one or more abilities within different channels. Objects which are at first visually perceived, for example, later become bonded to verbal abilities as labels are attached to them by the child. Visual shapes, which at first are perceived and discriminated, will later be drawn as bonds are formed between the perceptual and motor channels within the child's attribute pattern.

6. Some of these bonds are what might be termed *imperative*, relative to society's expectations, i.e. bonding between the visual appearance of word shapes, and their verbal-cognitive meanings.

7. Some bonds are rather specific and are due to environmental circumstances and conditions unique to an individual, as for example the bonds formed as the university student learns a new language, or the names the child of a naturalist may attach to birds he observes.

8. Not only do pairs and groups of abilities tend to become associated or bonded together as a function of maturation, but at a later time, abilities which were previously connected may become functionally rather independent again. It is not efficient for a child of four or five to watch his feet while he walks, while before the age of four, the functional connection between the sight of his feet (perceptual) and the feet movements (movement) was an important and necessary bond. As a child learns to read well, lip movements need not be paired with the cognitive representation of the word, just as adults can write their names and pick up water glasses without the necessity for direct visual inspection of these types of acts seen in younger children.

Implications for Educators

1. Educators should be sensitive to the manner in which normal maturation takes place, and just when and what number of abilities are likely to appear in the maturing child and youth.

2. Educators should also be sensitive to the manner in which a given child may evidence uneven development, relative to the four channels of abilities outlined. Children assigned to wheel chairs since birth need not necessarily be stunted intellectually;

some retardates have superior motor abilities, while clumsiness is not always a sign of poor reading ability or potential. The nature of a given child's attribute pattern, of course, emerges from a comprehensive testing program, uncontaminated by prior assumptions about purported relationships between different abilities.

3. At times educators need to provide an environment which will result in a child expanding his abilities within a given channel, or they may need to provide conditions which aid a child to form *imperative* functional bonds between two or more abilities. Writing training may be needed for a child who does not pair visual perceptual abilities and hand movements; while the numerous functional bonds which are needed in reading, between cognitive and visual-perceptual abilities, may need extra attention to be developed.

4. At other times educators may need to build synthetic bonds between abilities in order to circumvent various kinds of blunting which may be tested and observed. A central-city child for example, may lack the incentive to read well, while placing a high value upon physical activity. Thus, for example, one may build synthetic bonds between reading and physical activity by exposing the youngster to reading and spelling games in which he utilizes his physical capacities in vigorous ways.

Epilogue

There are other ways in which the model outlined may be considered. For example, it is assumed that various school district specialists should be thoroughly familiar with the manner in which a particular ability channel diffuses, proliferates, and ties into (bonds with) other channels. The language-speech specialist for example, should be thoroughly familiar with the verbal channel described, while the reading specialist should be cognizant of the manner in which both perceptual and cognitive abilities relate as the child matures. The physical education teacher should similarly be familiar with the way in which motor abilities emerge as the child matures.

Others in education may take upon themselves to become well-grounded in another side of the model; that is, individuals working with a particular age range would seem to have the obligation to become familiar with the manner in which a variety of abilities emerge and interrelate within a given maturational period. The first grade teacher, for example, should be aware of how speech and motor behaviors, as well as perceptual and cognitive behaviors emerge and integrate in the child of 5½ to 6½ years.

The model outlined in these brief paragraphs is not a simple one, as indeed it is believed that the maturational process is not simple. Rather it is an attempt to explain the unevenness seen in many children's ability patterns. Moreover it has been attempted to suggest how knowledge about maturational change in human abilities forms helpful guidelines for effective practices.

BIBLIOGRAPHY

1. Bousefield, Weston A.: Motor primacy and behavioral development. In Kuhlen, Raymond and Thompson, George: *Psychological Studies of Human Development.* New York, Appleton, 1970, pp. 116–125.
2. Clausen, John.: *Ability Structure and Subgroups in Mental Retardation.* Washington, Spartan, 1966.
3. Cratty, Bryant J.: *Perceptual and Motor Development in Infants and Children.* New York, Macmillan, 1970.
4. ———: *Physical Expressions of Intelligence.* Englewood Cliffs, P-H, 1972.
5. ———: *Human Behavior: Exploring Educational Processes.* Wolfe City, University Pr, 1971.
6. Fleishman, E.: Factorial analysis of complex psychomotor performance and related skills. *J Appl Psychol*, vol. 40, no. 2, 1956.
7. Garrett, H. E.: A developmental theory of intelligence. *Am Psychol,* 1:372–378, 1946.
8. Illingworth, R. S.: *Development of the Infant and Young Child.* Edinburgh and London, E & S Livingstone, 1967.
9. Meyers, C. E., and Dingman, H. F.: "The structure of abilities at the preschool ages: Hypothesized domains. *Psychol Bull*, 57:514–32, 1960.
10. Smith, Olin W.: Developmental studies of spatial judgments by children and adults. *Percept Mot Skills*, 22:3–73, Monograph, Supplement I-V22, 1966.

PART III

MODIFYING MOVEMENT ATTRIBUTES: THEORY, PROGNOSIS AND PRACTICE

CHAPTER 9

THE DEVELOPMENT OF THE BODY IMAGE: A MODEL*

An Overview

HISTORICALLY, concern for the improvement and habilitation of human movement capacities may be traced back to the writings of physicians from ancient China, India and Greece. For example, a series of ritualistic positions termed Kung Fu was prescribed by the Taoist priests of China 1,000 years before the birth of Christ; activities were intended to relieve pain and other symptoms. Physical exercises and spiritualistic experiences were combined in the temples of the early Greeks before the time of Homer, and gymnasia were annexed to many of these temples in order that beneficial exercises might be practiced. Throughout the centuries which followed varying amounts of attention were accorded exercise by the physicians of Europe, and Asia.†

It has only been within recent years that the term body-image has been employed in the literature, and during these recent decades it has taken on numerous definitions. Some of these concepts of the body-image have been connected more closely to the results of various kinds of physical exercise, while other writings have employed the hyphenated term body-image to denote more subtle perceptual awarenesses of the locations, functions, surfaces, and relationships of the body and its parts.

During the decades following World War II, the writings of

---

* Prepared for the Workshop For The Mentally Retarded at the Georgia Retardation Center, Atlanta, Georgia, held September 18th to 19th, 1973.

† A rather thorough look at the historical essay of therapeutic physical exercise may be found in the text edited by Sidney Licht, *Therapeutic Exercise*, (Baltimore, Waverly Press Inc., 1965).

numerous authors have further fanned the interest of laymen and professionals in interrelationships between the individual's psychological self, and various kinds of muscular experiences. These authors have included physicians, psychologists, paramedical therapists, educators, and at times quacks. The claims for the outcomes of various kinds of physical activity by these same individuals have ranged from the sensible and realizable, to the nonsensical, and mystical.

One of the outcomes of these writings has been the establishment of literally thousands of physical programs for children and adults, atypical and ordinary, which seem to recognize the relationships between sensory and motor processes, and between the physical reality and the individual's perceptions of his body. The content, objectives, as well as the "customers" of these programs vary widely—variances dependent upon geographical location and the needs of the local community, as well as upon the philosophical and educational backgrounds of the practitioners involved. This diversity is reflected in the labels given them by their instigators, names which range from sensory-motor education, perceptual-motor training, motor-sensory awareness, movement education, to body-awareness clinics, institutes for human potential, and on and on.

Moreover, the recipients of the attention of individuals working through the physical realm range from the blind, the multiply handicapped, the profoundly retarded, the emotionally disturbed and the severely brain damaged child and adult, to children and youth who may evidence only minor learning problems, or who may be free of any measurable physical, educational or psychological problems.

The objectives of these same programs also differ widely, and range from purposes which encompass a broad range of human attributes, to those which focus rather precisely upon measurable and observable physical problems. The location of these programs also varies, and they may be found in schools of general and special education, within the wards of state mental hospitals, resident schools for the blind and/or the retarded, and in the schools for the severely physically handicapped.

Despite the diversity of content, aims, and patients, these

programs have several common elements. For the most part they attempt to employ physical activities in direct or indirect ways. Secondly, the content, with few exceptions, involves activities which go on outside the individual's body. That is, the objective is to somehow modify functions by the application of techniques which are peripheral. The individuals involved do not have the frequent services of individuals qualified to engage in frequent corrective neurosurgery, or even those who might modify the biochemical make-up of the patients via the administration of medication. Since the middle of the 1960's during my visits to many of these programs I have been struck not only by the diversity alluded to, but also by the seemingly eclectic and pragmatic nature of the rationale underlying the selection of their content. Some sensory-motor educators seem to have attached themselves strongly and in exact ways to techniques outlined by some of the more prominent writers on the subject, while others have put together a broad range of activities, a selection which may be more or less successful depending upon the insight, background, and professional guidance of those in charge. It has further been my observation that positive results are more likely to be forthcoming when a reasonably broad range of activities is employed, by individuals whose professional backgrounds, and those of their frequent consultants, is broad and deep, than when the background of the practitioners is shallow, and when the range of activities is limited.

The primary purpose in constructing the model, which will be described, is to aid individuals believing in the worth of various kinds of sensory-motor, or perceptual-motor education, to perceive in rather broad terms what is available to them by way of therapeutic strategies, what functions and spatial dimensions of movement they may hope to positively effect, as well as the number of rather subtle objectives they may attain, or at least work toward. It is further hoped that the model to be described will offer some guidelines to researchers interested in relationships between movement activities and possible changes in physical as well as psychological characteristics. It is expected that the model may be of some assistance in the physical improvement of the multiply handicapped child and youth, of the blind, the retarded, as well as the severely or moderately brain damaged child, youth and adult. It should be emphasized at this point, that the model is not meant to be prescriptive, its guidelines *do not* contain suggestions for applications or techniques appropriate for a given child, or group of children. As was alluded to, the effectiveness of specific activities upon a child, or group of children, youth, or adults, depends upon the insights, and professional expertise of those administering and conducting the program.* The purposes of the model are to broaden perspectives, to help practitioners gain comprehensive perspectives of what may be available to them, and to aid them to expand the goals they might hold when using the physical components of the patient's personality as remedial tools.

Introduction

The model contains three major dimensions. These include (a) a coordinate labeled "therapeutic strategies," within which are contained some types of approaches which may be employed by a therapist-educator when working with movement as a method; (b) a second dimension named "dimensions of the proximal space field." Contained within this second coordinate are various compartments of space, within which the body, and its parts move, contact objects, and otherwise function. (c) The final dimension of the model contains what might be termed "perceptual-motor" goals. These objectives include the obvious as well as the subtle objectives which may be outcomes of a program of sensory-motor training and education.

(A) Therapeutic Strategies

Numerous therapeutic strategies have been employed throughout past as well as recent history, only some of which are listed within this first dimension of the model. Listed first are

---

* It should be further noted here, that the outcomes of a program of peripherally applied movement activities of various kinds to a given group of people are largely unpredictable. Cohen, as well as others, has conducted experiments with animals as well as humans, which point quite clearly to the wide variation present in the neuro-motor make-ups of several members of the animal kingdom, including man, variations which render uncertain the outcomes of assisted, resisted, or self-initiated movements.

assistive movements, in which the individual is helped by the therapist to engage in various actions. The methods of Kabat, as well as other prominent physical therapists, contain these types of activities, which may be accompanied by verbal reinforcement, explanation, and/or tactual activity.

Also listed are what are termed *resistive movements* in which the educator-therapist may resist the exertions of his patients, in rather total ways which would induce a static or isometric type of contraction; or the therapist may resist while permitting movement, resulting in what is termed an isotonic contraction on the part of the patient.

A third component within the dimension labeled "therapeutic strategies" has been termed "self-initiated movements," including efforts which the patient makes through his or her own volition, free from externally applied assistance or resistance. These movements may be initiated by the internalized volition of the patient himself, or because of stimulation and motivating conditions initiated by the therapist-educator. A child may simply extend his arm, for example, without the presence of an object to grasp, or the child may extend his arm because of the presence of an interesting object placed in proximity by the therapist-educator.

A fourth type of strategy has been named "tactual-stroking." The therapeutic methods proposed by Rood to deal with cerebral palsy emphasize this type of activity, as do the methods advanced by Jean Ayres, in an effort to overcome what she has termed "tactual defensiveness." These tactual activities may be encouraged by the therapist, as the patient strokes one hand with the other, or one foot passes along the opposite leg, or they may be initiated and administered by the therapist-educator. Other subdivisions of this therapeutic technique include one in which the limb, or body of the patient remains passive, while being stroked by a towel, or hand of the therapist-educator; as well as a second subdivision in which the patient makes some volitional effort to move himself or his limbs past some kind of immobile surface resulting in tactual input. An example of this latter technique would include rolling along the floor, with the back, sides, and front consecutively touching the floor's surface.

There are several other important and potentially helpful

types of therapeutic strategies. For example, the use of external bracing, is helpful in many cases of severe or moderate physical handicaps. Techniques expounded by the Bobaths, involving the release of reflexes, with accompanying assistive movements are important, and are explained in some detail in the text by Pearson and Williams.[8] Further sub-components of the "therapeutic strategies" dimension, include the use of various environments in which exercises may take place, including water, mud and the like. While it should be finally pointed out that most effective programs of physical rehabilitation and therapy contain a combination of approaches, indeed a given administration of a movement or exercise often combines several of these strategies. For example, when assisting movements, the therapist often affords the patient tactual input as the limb is held, while offering verbal accompaniment as the limb transcribes a pathway through space.

(B) Dimensions of the Proximal Space Field *

The second major dimension of our model involves the various compartments of space through which the body and its components may move, and may occupy. A consideration of these is important from a developmental as well as from a remedial standpoint. These compartments include those which the fingers and hands may occupy as they move. These, as well as the space in which the arms and legs move are described as "cones," as it is believed that if one examines the total movements of which the arms, legs, fingers, and hands are capable it will be noted that conelike space fields are involved, with the apex of the cones the joints from which the arms (shoulders), and fingers attach.

Developmentally, a child also begins to move his total body through various cylinders of space. As he learns to turn over, the cylinder occupied by his body and its parts is rather short, and its long axis is horizontal. And as he sits up, the cylinder of space he occupies is upright. These two space cylinders, a horizontal and vertical one, become elongated. As he moves from a sitting to a standing position he thus enlarges the vertical cylinder, and

---

* This concept was presented first in a text by the author, titled *Movement and Spacial Awareness in Blind Children and Youth*, Charles C. Thomas 1970, in a Chapter titled "The Body Image," Springfield, Illinois.

as he learns to crawl forward he lengthens the horizontal cylinder of space his body occupies. A "hallway of space" is occupied as the child learns to walk, a subdimension also indicated on the accompanying model. While whole compartments of space are opened up to the maturing child as he learns to navigate through his environment aided by an intact visual apparatus.

It should be emphasized here that this second dimension of our schema may be fully understood and exploited only if the therapist-educator obtains a thorough and clear-cut picture of the nature of normal perceptual-motor development. For when this picture is obtained, he or she may then structure and sequence experiences which follow in logical developmental order, from the easier, seen early in the life of the normal child, to the more complex seen later in the life of the normal child. That is, remedial techniques intended to enhance the movement and perceptual capacities of the atypical (whether child or adult) may be helpfully applied only to the extent to which the therapist-educator understands normality. The atypical, severely retarded adult, for example, may be encouraged to develop in ways similar to that of the normal child, i.e. learning to turn over, etc., in a manner, at a time of life, and at a pace highly dissimilar to the normal.

Finally, the "space field" dimension should include a subcomponent which involves a combination of spacial compartments. That is, a child may occupy more than one compartment of space at a given time, as he for example attempts to sit up, (this occupying a vertical cylinder of space) while attempting to manipulate an object with his hands and arms (contained in a cone of space directly to his front). Or he may be walking through a hallway of space, while attempting to retain his grasp upon an object contained within a space cone surrounding the hand-wrist region.

(C) Perceptual-Motor Goals, Objectives

Some of the objectives listed within this dimension are rather straightforward and obvious, while others are more subtle in nature. Among the latter are those perceptions which probably begin to emerge and develop well before the conscious memory of a normal child develops. These subtle objectives (i.e. that body parts have surfaces) are of vital importance, but are so remote from the earliest conscious memories of the therapists themselves that they are sometimes overlooked when formulating goals for programs for the atypical.

The first subdivision of this final dimension of our model is an obvious one. The child, youth, or adult must become aware of, and capable of exercising his movement capacities. Moreover these movements must be modifiable so that they may be made to vary in force and space when environmental requirements dictate. Additionally these movements, within each of the space compartments previously discussed, should be comprehensive, complete, consist of *all possible* movements of which the body, and/or its parts, together or singularly, are capable.

The second subdivision has been named gravitational relationships, and involves the sometimes obvious, and sometimes elusive, acquisition of perceptions which involve the orientation of the body, and/or its parts to gravity. The child must be able to balance well in a sitting position before arising to a standing position, for example; while even within the hand-arm space cones this gravitational objective is operative. It is not uncommon to observe the child with cerebral palsy, or the young normal child, hit himself in the eye with his hand as he reaches out to contact an object while lying on his back, and fails to perceive how gravity will pull his hand toward his face when he relaxes or contracts the wrong muscles. Gravitational relationships are also of course operative in the act of walking.

The third subdivision within our objective dimension is that the patient must be made aware of the fact that objects are located within the various spacial cones in which his body and/or its parts may be located. Additionally, the child or adult must be made to understand that both his body, and/or its parts cannot occupy, at the same time, space occupied by objects in close proximity. The early acquisition of this awareness is sometimes seen in the surprised look upon the face of the normal newborn as he suddenly and unexpectedly contacts an object held over his crib. It is obvious that this type of objective must be a major one when working with children, youth, and adults who are blind or have only partial vision. This subject is discussed at some length in a previous text by the author. Again, as in the case with all major dimensions of our model, the effective implementation and realization of this objective rest upon the therapist-educator's knowledge of the sequences of manipulative behavior developing in the normal child, from crude contacts to precise grasps and manipulations.

Another objective contained within this dimension is listed as "body-parts have surfaces." This objective may be reached, for the most part through the application of various kinds of tactual experiences. This type of awareness is seemingly more difficult to acquire in body parts and surfaces which are removed from the space field of the child or youth. Perceptual-motor therapists have spent a considerable amount of time designing activities and engaging in strategies intended to give the severely retarded child an awareness of his back, for example.

Learning that body parts have volume is another of the more subtle objectives, and may be acquired in conjunction with activities which involve manipulation and contact. The drawing of the child's body, and the subsequent inspection of the drawings also may give the child or youth some idea of his dimensions.

Further, it is obvious that a given activity or objective is not always worked for in isolation. A given activity (e.g. being wrapped in a mat while being stroked) may heighten the individual's awareness of the fact that his body has given volume, as well as an awareness that his body contains surfaces in various locations, and of various sizes.

Epilogue

The model as outlined may result in several types of activities on the part of the interested reader, including outright rejection. A helpful mental exercise, and one which is recommended for thorough understanding, is to try to decide just what kinds of activities may be represented by the interactions (within the small cubes which make up the larger spatial model) of the three major coordinates. For example one may take a goal (gravitational relationships), a dimension of the space field (walking hallway), as well as a strategy (self-initiated movement) and determine what kind of activities might be placed in the box at the point of their intersection. In this case line walking and/or balance beam walking is suggested.

Next the reverse operation may be explored. The reader may start with an activity observed in a program, and try to work backward, determining what objective(s) it apparently is pointed toward, what kind of therapeutic strategy it represents, and in addition what dimensions within the proximal spatial field of the individual seem to be occupied. After this operations-to-dimensions exercise has been attempted the reader may then try any of the following activities:

(A) A program in operation may be examined and evaluated, relative to the model, in an attempt to ask the following questions. What activities seem to correspond to the various objectives, strategies, and space dimensions contained in the model? What objectives seem to be ignored upon inspection of the program content? Are all of the objectives contained in the model, the therapeutic strategies etc., really appropriate for the type of patient served in the program? How might the program be expanded so as to include more available therapeutic strategies and objectives, if indeed such an expansion is desirable?

(B) A new program might be formulated with reference to the model. The program, hopefully preceded by a thorough evaluation of the prospective patients,* might align itself with various (or most) of the objectives shown, and might contain a selection of the therapeutic strategies presented.

(C) An ambitious researcher might search the literature to determine which strategies and program content seem most viable with reference to changes in abilities and perceptions contained in the model. An exercise of this type is likely to reveal that large programs of research are needed—explorations which should occupy the entire careers of more than one energetic young man or woman.

(D) The theoretically minded might further expand, modify, or otherwise adjust the model presented. The schema outlined is meant to be suggestive, and provocative, rather than prescriptive,

---

* Suggested evaluation tools are contained in the bibliography.

or absolute. Indeed the term model usually denotes a theory of which one is highly unsure, and indeed the author is far from certain of the viability of this one.

Finally it should be noted that the author has been highly impressed with the attempts made by many dedicated individuals to aid, help, change, and otherwise improve the lot of unfortunate children and adults through the use of sensory-motor activities. At times their energies have outstripped common sense, and even kindness; while at other times their efforts have been human, thorough and intelligent within limitations imposed by present knowledge of behaviorial change, neurology, and psy-

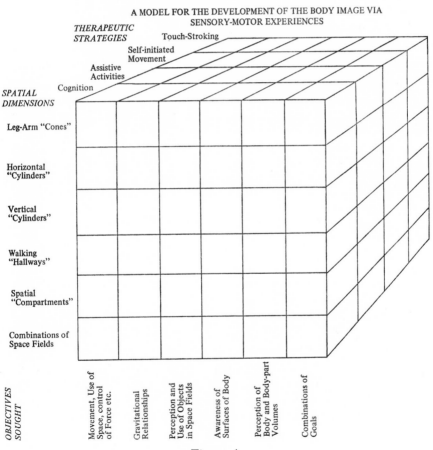

Figure 4.

EXAMPLES OF TECHNIQUES

SPATIAL COMPARTMENTS	TACTUAL STROKING	ASSISTIVE ACTIVITIES	SELF-INITIATED MOVEMENTS	
Finger cones	Rubbing fingers against another object and against each other	Moving fingers	Finger tapping by the blind child	Tactual exploration of shapes
Arm-leg cones	Stroking limbs, touching limbs to each other	Moving arms and legs through range of motion	Controlled movements of arms and legs	Reaching out to touch objects with feet and hands
Horizontal body cylinder	Stroking surfaces	Turning the infant in his crib	Rolling in crib or on the floor	Turning to grasp an object which touches back
The body's vertical cylinder	Standing within a padded tube, rolling around vertical tube	Assisting in support for crawling, in standing	Self-induced standing	Standing to reach sound and/or object above head
The body's crawling "tunnel"	Crawling along padded channel	Assisting in crawling	Self-initiated crawling	Crawling to reach sound and/or object
The body's walking "hallway"	Walking along narrow padded channel, touching sides with body	Assisting in walking	Self-initiated walking	Walking to reach sound and/or object goals

chology. It is hoped that the model described and depicted, will afford these energetic people some direction for their efforts, and will have some slight influence upon improving the quality of service they attempt to render to some of the more unfortunate members of society.

BIBLIOGRAPHY

1. Cohen, L. A.: Manipulation of cortical motor responses by peripheral sensory stimulation. *Arch Phys Med Rehabil,* 50:495–505, no. 9, September, 1969.
2. Cratty, B. J.: *Movement and Spatial Awareness in Blind Children and Youth.* Springfield, Thomas, 1970.
3. Cratty, B. J.: *Perceptual and Motor Development of Infants, and Children.* New York, Macmillan, 1970.
4. Cratty, B. J.: *Physical Activities for Children.* Freeport Long Island, Educational Activities Inc., 1974.
5. Cratty, B. J.: *Physical Expressions of Intelligence.* Englewood Cliffs, P-H, 1972.
6. Cratty, B. J., and Sams, T.: *The Body Image of Blind Children.* New York, American Foundation for the Blind, 1969, Monograph.
7. Licht, S. (Ed.): *Therapeutic Exercise.* Baltimore, Waverly Press, 1965.
8. Pearson, P. H., and Williams, C. E.: *Physical Therapy Services in the Developmental Disabilities.* Springfield, Thomas, 1972.

CHAPTER 10

PRINCIPLES OF PERCEPTUAL-MOTOR TRAINING FOR CHILDREN WITH MINIMAL NEUROLOGICAL HANDICAPS

Introduction

T HE VALUE OF an educational program can only be assessed indirectly, by measuring changes in the desired behaviors of the participants. Therefore to properly assess the effectiveness of educational programs for children with minimal perceptual-motor problems one must first ascertain what components of their motoric functioning are deficient, expose them to tasks which would seem to rectify these deficiencies and then retest them. Therefore our first job is to ascertain just what it is that these children can or cannot do, what interferes with their effective functioning in and with various components of their environment.

Fortunately two recent investigations using a combined total of about 150 neurologically handicapped children have been carried out, producing findings which begin to delineate the general and specific perceptual-motor deficits which should probably be attended to when planning a program.[1,3] Jean Ayres, in a factor analysis published in 1965, identified five general areas of perceptual-motor dysfunction as the result of exposing 100 children with suspected dysfunction to a battery of thirty-five tasks.

The factors identified include:

1. *Body Image Deficit:* reflected in tasks involving the ability to duplicate accurate bodily and hand movements, in tasks requiring the accurate localization of fingers, and in other tests of tactile perception. The factor loadings suggested that hand-finger image and body image are related attributes.

84

2. *Perceptual Dysfunction—Lack of Awareness of Form and Position in Two-Dimensional Space:* This factor involves scores on tests evaluating the perception of form and position in space, using both vision and tactile-kinesthetic cues without vision.
3. *Hyperactivity-Distractability:* Identified by tasks indicating a deficit in tactile perception accompanied by hyperactive behavior. (Evidence of attempts to escape the testing situation with verbal and motor behavior were one measure contributing to this factor).
4. *Integration of the Two Sides of the Body:* Tests of rhythm and of the proficiency with which a child crosses his body (or attempts to avoid doing so) contribute to this factor.
5. *Figure-Ground Discrimination:* The inability to select superimposed figures out of confused backgrounds, and similar tasks.
6. *Balance:* Obtained when tasks involving one-legged standing balance with eyes open and closed were analyzed.

While the majority of the tasks included in Ayres' thirty-five battery test differentiated significantly between the 100 neurologically handicapped children and a control group of fifty "normals," it is interesting to note that the tests of mixed dominance involving hand-eye use revealed that this purported symptom of perceptual disorganization was as prevalent within the normal population as within the experimental group. Another finding which questions common folklore involved the lack of relationship found between left-right discrimination on the body and left-right decisions in visual space.

This latter finding might be explained by the seeming differentiation between bodily tonus and visual judgments revealed in the study carried out in 1957. Exploring the sensory-tonic theory of perception developmentally, it was found that bodily tonus seemed less related to spatial judgments in late childhood than was seen when younger children's bodily tonus was altered with the accompanying request to make accurate estimates of verticality.[9]

The lack of congruence between the commonly held clinical assumption that cross-dominance accompanies neuromotor deficits reflected in learning problems may be explained by suggesting that such children simply accommodate to the inconvenience of dissimilar hand-eye preference, if indeed such a lack of hand-eye integration is really a critical problem at all.

In an investigation carried out in 1967 under the sponsorship of county, city, and state agencies, approximately fifty children were evaluated in a variety of perceptual-motor tasks within six categories. These children ranged in age from five to nineteen years and had been classified as educationally handicapped by the Los Angeles City Schools.[3] The findings of this study provide further guidelines for program planning.

It was found that only about one third evidenced atypical gait patterns while walking and crawling, although about two thirds failed to take a step with the proper foot when throwing. Moving backwards and laterally also proved difficult for these children, as did quickly arising from a back lying position on the mat.

In general, these children evidenced the most marked deficits in tasks involving the integration of movement with vision, including hand-eye, body-eye, or foot-eye coordination. Similar to the findings of Ayres, these data revealed that the children were unable to make various left-right discriminations about their body, with accuracy. The findings of the body-perception category suggested a sixteen step developmental sequence, which was later validated with a group of normal children at UCLA's University Elementary School.

The educationally handicapped children within the population studied exhibited motor competencies typical of well-functioning children from two to four years their juniors.

A striking finding with important implications for the early detection and alleviation of these perceptual-motor deficiencies was revealed when the data was inspected upon a developmental continuum. The best performance scores recorded by children were between the ages of eleven and twelve. After late childhood was reached, performance deteriorated. It might be hypothesized that as these children meet frustrations and failure when attempting to function motorically, they withdraw from situations in which such competencies are needed, and this withdrawal further lowers capacities. This may set in motion a relatively irrevocable cycle of failure, perceived ineptitude, withdrawal from participation, and lowering of capacity to perform further failure, etc.

The score on the best battery, most predictive of the total

battery score, was that obtained in the balance category. At the same time intercorrelations between the various qualities evaluated revealed that these children function in rather specific ways. These data thus suggest that programs for the neurologically handicapped child contain several kinds of activities, rather than relying upon one or two movement panaceas.

PROGRAM IMPLICATIONS

The findings presented above could have been recited by every parent of a neurologically handicapped child without the aid of test batteries, Ph.D.'s and complex computers. The critical questions in the minds of parents concern the components of programs for the amelioration of these subtle and obvious deficits. Parents become trapped by several kinds of circumstances when seeking help for their children: the rather ambiguous terms which are applied by the members of various disciplines whom they consult—complex jargon usually representing relatively simple behavioral manifestations; the difficulty of determining the relative influence of environmental, emotional and structural factors upon the behavior evidenced; the supposition on the part of some that perhaps the child's problem is only transitory or may be eliminated with some kind of movement panacea similar to the curing of an infection through the administration of an antibiotic; and, also by the variety of special schools, reading specialists, "educationalists," etc., who seem to be attracted to the *business* of *helping* children for reasons which are other than altruistic.

I believe programs for neurologically handicapped children should be based upon several principles. The components should be based upon the best experimental evidence available, rather than upon the blind acceptance of the unsubstantiated theoretical outpouring of some "Movement Messiah." The program should be under conditions which are motivating and relatively tension free. The program should involve exposure to a number of kinds of movement tasks encompassing those designed to enhance body-hand image; locomotor abilities; visual-motor integrations of hand-eye, body-eye, foot-eye; balance of various types (static and dynamic balancing); and those designed to lead toward useful classroom skills and socially desirable sport skills.

The diagram which follows contains two classifications: "Perceptual-Motor Categories" which involve various kinds of attributes which should be improved when possible, and "General Considerations." Although the list of "Perceptual-Motor Categories" contains eight constituents, this does not mean that all of these attributes should or can be incorporated into every program at a given time. Rather the instructor should attempt to select those which are appropriate to the assessed deficiencies of the children in his charge. It is also apparent that several of these categories overlap, and thus, a single activity might result in the improvement of more than one attribute.

Along the left-hand side of the following page are placed what has been termed "General Considerations." These are basic principles which should be attended to by those in charge and which underlie the performance of a variety of tasks. Within the squares in the center of the diagram are specific program suggestions, involving an integration of the attributes it is desired to improve with the "General Considerations" list on the right.

An important general consideration which has not been included on the charts involves what might be termed "Movement Differentiation." These kind of children frequently evidence the inability to direct their tensions and energies for a task in efficient and specific ways. Frequent residual tensions are often seen. A spillover of inappropriate tension in one arm, for example, is often seen as the child engages in an activity with the other. Upper body tension may accompany the child's efforts when jumping. Attempts to throw softly may be made in vain. Whenever possible the individual working with these children should be sensitive to this general and basic problem and should attempt to educate them to focus appropriate tensions in the body parts being utilized on the task at hand, and to differentiate between the body parts in use and those not involved directly.

The general considerations should be incorporated into the program as follows:

CONTROL. This implies that at times the child might be asked to move as slowly as he can, in an attempt to help him place him-

GUIDELINES FOR A PERCEPTUAL-MOTOR TRAINING PROGRAM FOR CHILDREN
WITH MINIMAL NEUROLOGICAL HANDICAPS

PERCEPTION-MOTOR → CATEGORIES	Body-Hand Image	Balance	Locomotion	Agility	Finger-Hand-Eye Interaction	Strength Endurance	Form and Movement Perception	Sport Skills
GENERAL CONSIDERATIONS Control	Slowly move your hand while watching it.	See how slowly you can walk the line	How slowly can you walk? How fast?	Can you stand up slowly?	How slowly can you draw a line?	Try fast push-ups and then a slow one	Trace around the figure slowly with your finger	Run-and-stop games
VISUAL-MOTOR PAIRING	Touch and look at your right hand with your left	Watch the moving point while standing	Jump into squares	Roll and look at a point up there	Place dots in the circles in time with the music	Sit up and look at the X, now down and see the other	Touch the ball swinging on the string as it passes you.	Let's play catch
Segmental Integrations	Move your left hand and right leg at once	Move down the beam using your arms to balance	Jump using proper arm action	Get up rapidly	Tap rhythmically with one hand twice and then the other	Hit with your left hand while shifting body weight	Trace a square with one hand and a circle with the other. Run and catch	Rebounding in basketball is like this!
Decision Shifting	How many left-right things can you do?	How many ways can you walk the line?	How many ways can you jump into the box?	How can you get up? Six ways?	How many ways can you draw a line from dot to dot?	Count and observe the form of his push-ups	How many ways can you bounce the ball?	Can you invent a game with a stick?
Social-Complexity	Touch your friend's right hand	Follow the leader down the beam	See how many ways your team can jump the line	Let's have a hi-jump contest	Bob, follow the line drawn by Jane on the board	Let's have a push-up contest	Bob . . . did Dick draw a triangle?	Now let's play with four on a side.

self under his own control. Vigorous and rapid activity, while called for at times, will many times merely further excite the already excitable youngster.

VISUAL-MOTOR PAIRING. When possible the child should be encouraged to involve visual control with his movements. Being asked to jump is not as productive as asking the child to jump with accuracy into a square, over a line, etc.

SEGMENTAL INTEGRATIONS. The activities in the program should encourage the child to integrate the various bodily segments, to involve the top of his body with the bottom, and one side with the other. For example, proper arm involvement should be encouraged when jumping, and proper bilateral arm involvement should be encouraged to aid in left-right integration.

DECISION SHIFTING. In line with "Control" above, the child, when feasible, should be permitted to make decisions relative to the task, evaluation, etc. The theoretical framework presented by Mosston outlines in detail how this may be accomplished using perceptual-motor activities as a learning modality.[5]

SOCIAL COMPLEXITY. Performance should be encouraged under conditions which gradually increase the complexity of social interactions and social stress. The child attempting to throw a ball to an adult therapist in an otherwise empty gymnasium is not comparable to playing catch with one's peers with the accompanying social punishment which may be received as the ball is dropped.[5]

It has not been attempted to outline exact developmental sequences designed to enhance these attributes. At the same time, it is believed that cognizance of these perceptual-motor categories and the manner in which they interact with "General Considerations" should provide sound guidelines for the development of programs containing the relatively unsophisticated tasks a child with a minimal neurological handicap truly needs.

BIBLIOGRAPHY

1. Ayres, Jean: Patterns of perceptual-motor dysfunction in children: A factor analytic study. *Percept Mot Skills,* Monograph Supplement 1–V20, 1965, pp. 335–368.

2. Cratty, Bryant J.: *Developmental Sequences of Perceptual-Motor Tasks.* Baldwin, Educational Activities, 1967.

3. ———: *The Perceptual-Motor Attributes of Mentally Retarded Children and Youth.* In cooperation with the Mental Retardation Services Board of Los Angeles County, August, 1966.

4. ———: *Movement Behavior and Motor Learning,* 2nd ed. Philadelphia, Lea & Febiger, 1967.

5. ———: *Social Dimensions of Physical Activity.* Englewood Cliffs, P-H, 1967.

6. ———: *Psychology and Physical Activity.* Englewood Cliffs, P-H, 1968.

7. ———: *Perceptual-Motor Behavior and Educational Processes.* Springfield, Thomas, 1964.

8. Delacato, Carl H.: *The Diagnosis and Treatment of Speech and Reading Problems.* Springfield, Thomas, 1964.

9. Mosston, Muska: *Teaching Physical Education.* Columbus, Merrill, 1966.

10. Wapner, S., and Werner, Heinz: *Perceptual Development, An Investigation Within the Framework of Sensory-tonic Theory.* Clark Pr. Dubuque, Iowa, 1957.

THE CLUMSY CHILD SYNDROME:
SOME ANSWERS TO QUESTIONS
PARENTS ASK

INTRODUCTION

During the past twelve years, a program was conducted at UCLA for the remediation of children with minor to moderate motor problems. The children are evaluated using a number of tests to assess their control of big muscles, their writing behavior, as well as their self-concept and game choices. While the children are being individually tested, the parents and the testing agent observe, using a one-way mirror arrangement, during this period of time. Afterward, the purposes of the testing are explained and the test results interpreted to the parents.

As these observations are being carried out, there are a number of questions which are frequently directed toward me. Indeed, one can identify from ten to twelve questions which occur with such regularity that it prompted the writing of the short monograph which follows. Such questions range from relatively simple pragmatic ones, revolving around programs of activity and remediation, to other more complex ones delving into causes of motor disturbances which, in order to be properly answered, require the expertise of a committee of neurologists, pediatricians, psychiatrists, and child psychologists. Indeed, a better subtitle for this publication might be *Some Tentative Answers to Questions Parents Ask*.

With these types of limitations in mind, the author will first state the question commonly asked and then briefly outline the type of answer usually formulated. It should be remembered that when considering these answers, they may not really be appropriate for the coordination problems of *your* child. Only a complete evaluation of a child's total emotional, social, academic, perceptual and motor abilities can truly serve his or her needs and result in the answers to specific problems which are best rendered by professionals qualified to diagnose and assess the various facets of his or her personality.

QUESTIONS AND ANSWERS

1. *Why is he this way? Why is he clumsy?*

There are numerous possible causes for minor to moderate movement problems in children ranging from difficulties encountered at birth due to heredity, emotional maladjustment, and early childhood diseases. Only your pediatrician can assign a reasonably accurate cause to a child's problem, but it is sometimes not as helpful if the parent dwells excessively on causes but rather looks carefully at the types of problems seen, such as hand-eye coordination in writing, balance and agility problems on the playground, running and walking awkwardly, and so forth, and then formulates a program which is intended to remediate these problems.

2. *My child reads well and is intelligent. Why does he have coordination problems?*

The nervous system is extremely complex, and often children are adequate or above average in verbal and reading comprehension and yet have coordination problems. We work each year with children from a school for the gifted who evidence motor development several years below that expected for children their age. It is true, however, that many clumsy children have difficulty expressing their intellect in handwriting, in finishing their math problems, in their spelling lesson, etc. Thus incoordination in writing provides a severe block to the expression of their intellect.

While it is generally true that there is a greater percentage of children with coordination problems among groups of children with learning problems including reading, there are children who are adroit at games and yet have learning difficulties for a variety of reasons. There is also a considerable amount of research in literature confirming the fact that basic programs of movement activities will not necessarily aid reading in either the poor reader or average reader.

3. *But can my child be made better? Can he be changed?*

Our research indicated that the children most likely to change include those who are younger, from two to six years of age, as well as those whose motor problems are less marked. Most likely to change are measures of a child's fitness and strength; next liable to change are measures of coordination, balance, agility, throwing and the like; in questionnaires measuring the child's self-concept and collected by asking the child various questions (e.g. "Are you the last to be chosen in games?"), it is indicated that these feelings are more difficult to modify quickly than are his physical performance scores.

4. *How long will it take to improve his coordination?*

Motor incoordination is not an infectious disease which is checked via a quick inoculation of some kind of movement panacea. Children in the program at UCLA are not retested until they have participated about six months. When and if a child's motor competencies are helped to change, it is not clear whether some basic ingredient in his nervous system has been modified or whether he has simply been aided to develop more effective strategies when performing motor skills, such as standing with his feet further apart when throwing in the case of a balance problem, etc.

5. *What about little league, the program at the YMCA, and similar youth programs?*

The primary principle to keep in mind is that exposing a clumsy child to a program of physical activity is likely *never* to have a *neutral* effect upon his personality. It can be negative, indeed devastating, or emotionally uplifting, depending upon the philosophy, expertise, and patience of the instructor and the demands placed upon the child for quick improvement. It is important that before placing a child in such a program the parent observe the manner in which the instructor works with children and also spend time asking the instructor what he expects as well as telling him the child's problem. If the instructor is too demanding, the program too "high-powered" with relationship to the demands for excellence, the child with movement problems should be kept out of it. On the other hand, if the program is geared to the individual physical and emotional needs of the children participating, incorporates basically sound principles of teaching and learning, and contains adequate conditioning for strenuous activity, the child might be placed in it.

6. *What can I do with my child at home?*

Some parents can work with their own children in a program of remediation and some can not. If the child evidences problems of big muscle control, he might be given a program about three times a week (Monday-Wednesday-Friday) for an hour or less each time consisting of basic activities, including tumbling, balance beam work, some physical exercises, plus playground sport skills. The other days of the week (Tuesday-Thursday-Saturday) he might be given help with handwriting and printing.

There are a number of guides and booklets usable by parents containing helpful techniques, including those listed in the bibliography.[2,3,7] There are several general principles to follow:

(a) Work on simple tasks at first such as jumping over a line in various ways, moving laterally backward, and the like, before going to more complex tasks like running and catching balls thrown from a distance.

(b) Keep the practice as free from emotional stress as possible; encourage work within the child's capacities while attempting at times to help him to try to better his previously best efforts. Keep other children away who might ridicule his attempts at improvement.

(c) Work specifically on the areas of incompetence exhibited by the child; walking balance beams will help balance, not handwriting, for example. For help with the latter try practice in writing and printing using simple lead-up activities.

(d) Work both on basic activities such as agility, balance, and specific playground skills that the child says he needs. Ask "What are you doing in school now that I can help you with?" and then provide him with the activities he outlines.

(e) Provide a means following vigorous activity, through which the child can be aided to calm down. Relaxation training in which the child is placed in a comfortable position and then aided to alternately tighten and relax his muscles in response to your verbal commands, is a helpful activity, for example. Attempting to somehow drain off excess energy through vigorous physical activity when directed toward physically inept, hyperactive youngsters is likely to have a negative effect; they are likely to become overaroused and too upset to even sleep at night following the program to which they have been exposed.

A simple home gymnasium can consist of a 2″ x 4″ board ten to fifteen feet long in the back yard, a few balls, ropes and sticks to jump over. Most important is the creativity of the parent in utilizing these simple pieces of equipment. After closely directed activities are engaged in for a period of time ("Walk the balance beam as I show you"), children may be encouraged to demonstrate modifications of the activities to which they are exposed ("Jump over the line six different ways," or perhaps "Get from here to there four different ways").

I have recently seen some marvelous examples of children who have been aided by their parents, and have obviously been exposed to patience and kindness while being helped, and whose motor coordination has improved remarkably. On the other hand, special help might be sought, as the following answer indicates.

7. *Where can I receive help with my child?*

Hopefully, in the near future, all elementary and secondary schools will contain special remedial programs in which from 15 to 18 per cent of the children in these schools who are likely to exhibit motor problems are given help. In the meantime, there are often programs at the local college or university; a parent might call the physical education departments or the departments of psychology or special education. Such calls may help initiate a program where none now exists, by demonstrating need. Sometimes a group of parents can get together, hire a physical education instructor or college student, and obtain materials and the help of professional consultants who might direct their efforts.

There are a number of self-styled, perceptual-motor trainers in many communities today who may be evaluated using the following continuum: Do their credentials consist of mere interest, or do they have a background in education, special education, psychology and/or physical education? Do they promise to remediate all the child's educational, perceptual and emotional problems through motor activity? If they do, one should be extremely wary of working with them. Perhaps the family pediatrician or school psychologist can recommend someone who is professionally qualified to engage in a physical education program specially suited to the needs of the child.

8. *Won't he simply grow out of his coordination problems?*

The child may or may not; in any case it is believed imperative if the child is younger to expose him to some attempt at remediation. A number of children viewed in late childhood have been kept away from any early help, because of the "he'll grow out of it" philosophy. Usually, the emotional make-up seen in such children is extremely unstable, as they have received a number of years of social punishment from their peers by this time, and may also have incurred the censure of their teachers for failure to do their work in time.

9. *What can I do about the amount of special punishment heaped upon my child on the playground, because of his physical deficiencies?*

This is an extremely difficult problem. Most of the boys and girls tested report that their friends make fun of them, and in other ways direct ridicule toward them. Often an increase in skills elicits more favor from a child's classmates, but even improvement in physical skill frequently is not enough to overcome a reputation previously earned for clumsiness. Often a parent must remove a child from one school environment and place him in another, in order for him to exhibit his newly acquired physical skills.

Inordinate pressure from classroom teachers and/or physical education teachers for physical performance which the child is incapable of, should be treated by going to the teacher or principal and explaining the child's problem. If this is not effective, he might be removed from the school. Or perhaps a phone call from a professional worker (psychologist or physician) explaining the nature of the child's problem to the school official concerned might be helpful.

This type of social punishment is of course likely to compound the child's problem, and unless it is lessened, is likely to result in moderate to severe emotional problems. Without being overprotective, the parents should avail themselves of every means possible to prevent or lessen the impact or ridicule from other children or from school personnel. Fortunately, a great many school teachers and administrators in increasing numbers are sensitive observers of clumsy children and are instituting school programs to remediate this problem in the population for which they are responsible.

10. *Is this problem more prevalent in boys than in girls?*

Yes, it would seem so, and no one at this point seems to know the exact reasons why. At the same time it is becoming increasingly evident at UCLA that a clumsy girl often suffers social problems for her physical ineptitude similar to those experienced by clumsy boys.

11. *May the better feelings which a child will engender about himself when improving his physical ability and acquiring success in games reflect in improved school work?*

Sometimes improved self-concept will result in more effort in school work by a child and sometimes not. At times low ability and motivation in games are part of a general syndrome of effortlessness seen in a number of areas, a syndrome which should be explored in depth by a child psychologist or child psychiatrist. At other times we have seen marked improvement in self-concept acquired because of improved physical ability which then results in improved work in school. At other times, a child's improvement in sports may not generalize and the child still may feel badly about his academic progress and remain a low achiever.

12. *What about special lessons in an individual sport, tennis or swimming, for example? Will accomplishment in these activities through extra tutoring help a child?*

If the instructor is patient, and the group pressures not great, this kind of experience can help a child gain self-confidence through physical activity. Often these tutored games and activities are not those valued by his peers on the playground, and while swimming is an excellent conditioner and recreational activity, the transfer from swimming to other physical education activities seen on playgrounds is likely to be slight or absent.

13. *Will music lessons help or hinder a child?*

Again, if taught in a patient manner with little pressure, lessons in the piano, guitar, etc., may be helpful and enjoyable for a child with coordination problems. However, finger dexterity exercises, as seen in piano playing and guitar, etc., are not likely to help handwriting which employs a different type of coordination.

14. *How can I help my child's writing?*

Primarily by stress-free, short practice sessions at home using various materials prepared for this purpose, a child's writing can be improved. At the same time, some older children (10 and over) with coordination problems, can be aided to express their intellect by teaching them to type. Although typing requires a different kind of coordination than the more fluid writing and printing tasks, at times a child may be more proficient in the former than in the latter.

If a child's printing is extremely erratic his hand may have to be guided, with the parent sitting behind the child, in the formation of his letters. When more proficiency is achieved, a cookie pan, with about ¼ inch of modeling clay may be used as a surface for printing. Thus the clay guides the point of the writing implement to some degree. Later the child can trace over letters, and finally he may be able to print without help or visual guides.

15. *What is easier, cursive handwriting or block printing? Which should he try to do first?*

Many cursive letters, the l's, e's, and i's, for example, are similar to the early developmental stages in scribbling, and thus are probably easier for most children than the stop and go motions needed in printing. At the same time there are other written letters, most of the capital letters, and those requiring cut-backs, such as b, d, q, p, etc., which are probably more difficult for a child to execute than most of the printed letters. Cursive letters, or handwriting, prevent the reversals some times seen when letters are printed.

16. *What about letter reversals when my child prints?*

Reversing letters, and the order of letters in words, is typical of the normal five-year-old, just as the lack of accurate left-right awareness at this age, is common. Almost one half of all six-year-olds will occasionally reverse letters. By the age of seven or eight, however, this problem should disappear. Playing left-right games of various kinds with the child may help, particularly if, when a child is seated in front of letters and words, direct transfer instructions to the asymmetries of words and letters are taught (for example: "See Johnny, the curved part of the d faces toward your left hand"). However, the causes of poor reading are more complicated than simply reversal problems, and clearing up reversal problems will not always result in reading problems similarly disappearing.

17. Just what should a child be able to do with his body at various ages?

A paperback text listed in the bibliography [5] contains detailed guidelines. But, in general, by four years of age a normal walking and running pattern should be seen in children, and they should be able to walk two-inch wide lines on the floor without much trouble. By four and five, a child should be able to catch a large playground ball bounced to him from a short distance away, and should hop on one foot and jump using both feet at the same time for a short distance. If a child evidences problems executing these simple tasks, and in drawing reasonably good circles and squares by the time he enters school, it is possible that he is encountering some kind of problem using his body in various ways, and should be thoroughly evaluated by an educational psychologist and/or his doctor.

SUMMARY

Children with coordination difficulties are frequently found in so-called normal populations of children and consist primarily of boys. Remediation of their problems depends upon the age at which the problem is identified and the degree of dysfunction the child may evidence. Remedial measures should be properly sequenced and patiently applied, and should encompass a broad range of activities directed toward the child's specific coordination problems.

Such children should not be subjected to inordinately stressful physical education or athletic programs in which performance is emphasized, within emotionally charged conditions. Rather, they should be confronted with patiently applied physical activities in which they have some chance to do well. Handwriting and printing practice for short periods each day may result in improvement, just as should programs in which fitness and the control of the larger muscles of the body are emphasized.

The research literature is clear in substantiating the fact that improvement in motor coordination *will not* necessarily result in improvement in various visual perceptual abilities, or in reading proficiency. At the same time, a child who may be failing because of a low self-concept caused by the social punishment of his peers due to a lack of game proficiency may be helped in rather general ways by improving his coordination. Programs of remedial physical activities are important in achieving the goals inherent in the program, such as improving motor coordination without needing additional justification with reference to improvement in academic abilities.

BIBLIOGRAPHY

1. Blake, O. William and Volp, Anne M.: *Lead-Up Games to Team Sports*. Englewood Cliffs, P-H, 1964.
2. Cratty, Bryant J.: *Developmental Sequences of Perceptual-Motor Tasks for Neurologically Handicapped and Retarded Children*. Freeport, Lang Island, Educational Activities, 1967.
3. Cratty, Bryant J.: *Learning and Playing: Fifty Vigorous Activities for the Atypical Child*. Freeport, Long Island, Educational Activities, 1968.
4. Cratty, Bryant J.: *Trampoline Activities for Atypical Children*. Palo Alto, Peek Publications, 1969.
5. Cratty, Bryant J.: *Perceptual and Motor Development of Infants and Children*. New York, Macmillan, 1970.
6. Cratty, Bryant J.: *Active Learning*. Englewood Cliffs, P-H, 1971.
7. Cratty, B. J.: *Physical Activities for Children*. Baldwin, Educational Activities, 1973. (200 cards combining a wide range of motor activities intended to remediate the clumsy child.)
8. Cratty, Bryant J. and Martin, Sister Margaret Mary: *Perceptual-Motor Efficiency in Children, the Measurement and Improvement of Movement Attributes*. Philadelphia, Lea & Febiger, 1969.
9. Frostig, Marianne: *Movement and Education*. Chicago, Follet, 1970.
10. Humphrey, James, and Sullivan, Dorothy: *Teaching Slow Learners Through Active Games*. Springfield, Thomas, 1970.
11. Mosston, Muska: *Developmental Movement*. Columbus, Merrill, 1965.
12. Wallis, Earl L., and Logan, Gene: *Exercise for Children*. Englewood Cliffs, P-H, 1966.

MOVEMENT IN PROGRAMS FOR
HANDICAPPED CHILDREN: HYSTERIA
AND REALITY*

SINCE THE PUBLICATION of the texts by Strauss and Lehtinen, Getman and Kephart in the late 1940's and early 1950's, there has been an onrushing interest in the use of movement activities for the handicapped, unparalleled in the history of special education. Professionals, semiprofessionals and downright unprofessionals of a wide variety began to prescribe movement education programs containing a wide diversity of tasks, and these programs in turn were proposed for the remediation of many kinds of abilities in children and youth evidencing a wide range of problems.

The onrush of movement prescriptions for the correction of perceptual, visual, intellectual and academic problems was widely appealing for many reasons. Parents, sometimes for the first time, could become involved in helping their unfortunate children. Teachers whose minds were beginning to become rather boggled with the plethora of often subtle educational curealls, were handed rather obvious and easily understandable action cures, consisting of balance beam walking and the like. Children seemed to take to the sometimes funfilled activity programs, sessions of movement experiences which provided a needed break from often oppressive and physically confining sessions of traditionally applied academia.

Those who were convinced reached hard and long for various

---

* Outline of Dinner Speech, Conference on Physical Education Techniques and Methods for Handicapped Children and Youth, May 24, 1973.

perceptual-motor programs, either accepting intact the writings and content proposed by one of the "ordained," or else attempting to combine the best components contained in various authors' writings, in order to compile an ideal program for youngsters evidencing various problems.

But, amid the hysteria of the 1950's, 1960's and early 1970's, some discordant notes occasionally issued forth. For example, the admonition that "movement was the basis of the intellect" fell on puzzled ears of the parents of intelligent children afflicted with cerebral palsy. Could their children be academically incapable because they lacked movement capacities, they asked? Writers and theoreticians who proclaimed that sound intellectual and academic functioning was only possible if a child evidenced adequate movement abilities,* were somewhat puzzled at times to find clumsy children within schools for the gifted, or to observe physically superior retardates in the Special Olympics Programs sponsored by the Joseph P. Kennedy Jr. Foundation.

Most disturbing to the more sophisticated examiners of the passing movement scene, were the rather consistent research findings which indicated that the application *of a few simple movement* cures were not only highly unlikely to modify any academic or perceptual abilities, but also would not modify movement abilities. Following the negative research findings which poured forth, came official statements further reflecting skepticism, from such organizations as the American Academy of Pediatrics, the American Medical Association, the National Association for Retarded Children and similar groups interested in the welfare of the more unfortunate members of our youthful society.

Examination of the various movement theories and practices expounded during the 1950's and 1960's, also brought forth some guidelines and findings which if adhered to when further program development is engaged in, should help to replace movement hysteria with achievable realities. Some of the realities

---

* A movement expert in the San Fernando Valley last year proclaimed that no child should be admitted to elementary school unless he could skip: a perhaps useful criteria, as its application would eliminate the kindergarten and most of the first grade!

which I believe have been documented in the literature are as follows:

1. Movement is one of several important components of the child's emerging personality, not a central core from which all social, intellectual, perceptual and academic skills must invariably spring.

2. Clumsiness in children, whether academically gifted or possessing learning difficulties, poses social obstacles which must be overcome. With exposure to a broadly based program of movement experiences, it is likely to elicit some improvements in movement abilities.

3. A comprehensive program containing a wide variety of sensory-motor experiences has been shown to exert positive changes in some severely and profoundly retarded children. Due to individual differences in neuromotor makeup among these children, as well as among all children, the changes are likely to vary from child to child, exposed to the same program experiences.

4. Adequate hand-eye coordination is a necessary component of classroom functioning, enabling a child, whether gifted, average or below average academically, to answer questions and problems in written form and to express himself intellectually. Hand-eye coordinations involved in printing and writing tasks can often be improved by exposure to properly sequenced exercises.

5. Such academic operations as reading consist of numerous subprocesses, any one or combination of which if not in tact will likely impede progress. While most reading processes *may* be translated to movement experiences, they need not necessarily be.

6. A wide variety and combination of peripheral processes may be intact and/or deficit in various ways, while basic intellectual functioning may be relatively unimpaired. The way to change central intellectual processes is not by mindlessly applied peripheral movement and sensory experiences, but by involving the central processes directly, by encouraging the child to engage in all dimensions of intellectual behavior within a motivating program of movement experiences.

7. To an increased degree it has been found that when a

program of movement experiences is filled with academic content and/or *requires a child to think*, to make decisions about the learning process, and to engage in various intellectual operations, it is likely that such a program will exert a positive influence upon both academic competencies, as well as intellectual functioning. Programs of this nature should proceed along two main dimensions: On one hand, they should afford the child increased freedom to make at least some of the decisions about what he is undertaking, and secondly situations, and movement and action problems should be presented which contain increased difficulty, as the child evidences the ability to engage in the simpler intellectual operations.

Essentially, therefore, the research tells us that we cannot expect too much in what learning theorists call "transfer width." Transfer from program content to objectives is likely to take place *only* if the content of the program contains experiences which are compatible with stated objectives. A program containing a few simple movement experiences is likely to modify only those movement qualities contained in the actions presented and little else. Whereas, a program of action experiences in which children are required to make perceptual judgments, to create, to make decisions, to memorize and to use their intellectual abilities within many dimensions is likely to positively influence a wide variety of abilities.

The viable research literature over the past twenty-six years has informed us that movement experiences are potentially powerful tools. If these tools are properly sharpened, aimed and combined in reasonable ways, our contributions as physical educators and special educators are likely to be helpful ones in the lives of the children we hope to serve.

BIBLIOGRAPHY

1. Cratty, B. J.: *Physical Expressions of Intelligence*. Englewood Cliffs, P-H, 1972.
2. ———: *Intelligence in Action*. Englewood Cliffs, P-H, 1973.
3. ———: *Active Learning. Englewood Cliffs*, P-H, 1972.
4. ———: *Perceptual and Motor Development of Infants and Children*. New York, Macmillan, 1970.

5. Getman, G. N.: *How to Develop Your Child's Intelligence.* Luverne, A Research Publication, G. N. Getman, 1952.
6. Kephart, Newell C.: *The Slow Learner in the Classroom.* Columbus, Merrill, 1956.
7. Strauss, A. A. and Lehtinen, L. E.: *Psychopathology and the Education of the Brain Injured Child.* New York, Grune, 1947, vol. I, Fundamentals and Treatment.

CHILDREN WITH MINIMAL BRAIN DAMAGE: PROGNOSIS FOR THE REMEDIATION OF MOTOR PROBLEMS*

THERE HAS BEEN, within the past twenty-five years, as this group is aware, a considerable amount of interest surrounding the use of movement experiences with the brain injured youngster. While at times this interest has led to some rather bizarre theorizing and even more hysterically applied movement remedies, a positive outcome has been the attention drawn to children with minimal motor problems. Research indicates that from 15 to 18 per cent of all children consigned to an elementary school for normal youngsters evidence signs of motor discoordination which has some kind of neurological dysfunction at its root. This percentage is even higher in groups of children with learning disabilities and in schools for the retarded.

In 1961 a program was begun in Santa Monica, California, with the intent to explore the remediation of motor problems among children evidencing what was labeled as the "Clumsy Child Syndrome." This program has continued to the time of this writing and has at several points been accompanied by research in efforts to gain deeper understanding of the effects of program content upon the abilities of the children dealt with then and currently.

The children are referred to the program from a variety of sources, including the Department of Pediatrics, and Psychiatry,

---

* Presented to the American Psychological Association Convention on the panel titled "Evaluation of Learning in the Brain Injured," at Honolulu, Hawaii, September, 1972.

in the UCLA Medical Center, private pediatricians, and pediatric neurologists, as well as school psychologists, teachers, and parents. As would be expected the majority are boys; only about 20 to 30 per cent of those evaluated are girls.

During an initial hour-long testing session the children are exposed to a six-category test of gross motor functioning, the first part of the Frostig, as well as a self-concept test and a games choice test, together with other tasks designed for the subjective evaluation of motor function. Examples of these latter exercises include alternate hopping, lateral movement of the total body, finger opposition, as well as running behavior. This evaluation, which is observed by the parents and myself, is followed by a conference illuminating salient points observed during the testing period.

The children then usually participate in classes which meet twice a week, lasting about an hour at each session. In groups of four the children are exposed to tasks which represent areas of deficiency previously evaluated during an hour-long testing session at UCLA. The age-range with which we normally work includes four- to twelve-year-olds.

Basic principles followed include attempting to expose children to what is termed a "stress-success" cluster of tasks, i.e. tasks which both are taxing but able to be performed, as well as some which are stressful to a slight degree. Moreover, we try to gradually modify the amount of social stress imposed on the children by modifying the constitution and/or size of the group in which they are working. Graduated sequences of fine motor control tasks have been found helpful in changing handwriting and printing performance; while overall, as the children grow older, more and more sports skills are phased into a program which, for the younger ones, consist primarily of basic developmental activities, involving balance, agility and the like.[8]

As the result of our research and observations, the following picture is emerging:

(A) Most amenable to change are children who are younger, and whose problems are slight. There does not seem to be any significant sex differences in prognosis for change of motor problems.[7]

(B) Over the years approximately 80 per cent of the children referred to us are boys.

(C) As a group, boys afflicted with motor problems give answers reflecting lack of social acceptance on a standardized test of self-concept.[7]

(D) Easiest to change are qualities reflecting physical fitness. Next in order of difficulty are motor qualities involving accuracy and control, i.e. balance, agility, ball handling ability and the like. Most difficult to change, after five- to six-month period, are answers on the children's self-concept test.

(E) Little transfer will occur between training in fine motor qualities and those involving large muscle control. This finding prompted us several years ago to concentrate either on fine or gross motor problems, while working out a home training program for the quality not dealt with in the formal program.

(F) Hand-eye control is improvable not only with the application of remedial measures involving practice, but is also improved in hyperactive children with the application of medication.

(G) Improvement in groups of children exposed to a two-hour a week program of motor remediation will occur about three times more during a six-month period, in tests reflecting balance, agility and the like, than would be expected as the result of normal maturational changes.[7]

(H) A program of gross motor activities, if directional concepts are emphasized (i.e. jump up, more toward your right, etc.), results, after a five-month period, in significant improvement in a drawing test in which arrangement of figures in proper locations around the corners of a large square is required.[7]

(I) A group of boys with motor problems will evidence game-choice profiles similar to those of girls, while they will also tend to report playing games involving "fantasy bravery" (cops and robbers, spacemen, etc.) at older ages than do comparable boys, free of motor problems.[7]

(J) There are marked individual differences, as is usually found in programs of motor remediation, relative to susceptibility to remedial efforts. Cohen, among others, discovering differences in cortical responses following similar kinds of peripheral sensory stimulation, has concluded that unique patterns of inter-action between cerebral motor activity and peripheral sensory activity, within each individual, explain the differential success of various methods of remediation.[3]

(K) It is unclear whether changes recorded on tests are re-flective of basic neurological modifications to the demands placed upon the children, or whether they are simply due to the adoption of new and more effective strategies when attempting to accomplish motor tasks.

Our future research revolves around discovering the nature of the diffusion of ability patterns in children as a function of age. Thus, a hypothesis is being pursued similar to that espoused in 1946 by Garrett,[11] and since corroborated in recent studies relative to intellectual abilities.[10,12] Further investigations are exploring the nature of impulse control measures and their relationship to academic learning and I.Q. scores.[13,14] Moreover, following a four-year study of the effect of learning games on academic abilities in the central city of Los Angeles (Catholic Archdiocese), a program is being pursued to hopefully elicit change in certain intellectual attributes through selected, structured, and cognitively loaded programs of movement education, to which retarded children will be exposed.[9] The further illumination of racial differences in motor ability traits[1] and in self-control measures,[2] uncovered by several of our students, presents, other important directions for future studies.

BIBLIOGRAPHY

1. Bonds, Robert S.: A comparison of movement abilities exhibited by Chicano, white and black children. Unpublished, Perceptual-Motor Learning Laboratory, UCLA, 1971.
2. Burke, K.: A survey of selected self-control measures in elementary school children. Unpublished study, Perceptual-Motor Learning Laboratory, UCLA, 1970.
3. Cohen, L. A.: Manipulation of cortical motor responses by peripheral sensory stimulation. *Arch Phys Med. Rehabil*, 50:495–505, no. 9, September, 1969.
4. Cratty, B. J.: *Active Learning.* Englewood Cliffs, P-H, 1971.
5. ————: *Perceptual and Motor Development of Infants and Children.* New York, Macmillan, 1970.

6. ———: *Physical Expressions of Intelligence.* Englewood Cliffs, P-H, 1972.
7. Cratty, B. J., Martin, Sister M. M., Jannett, C., Ikeda, M., and Morris, M.: *Movement Activities, Motor Ability and the Education of Children.* Springfield, Thomas, 1970.
8. Cratty, B. J., Martin, Sister M. M.: *Perceptual-Motor Efficiency in Children: The Measurement and Improvement of Movement Attributes.* Philadelphia, Lea & Febiger, 1969.
9. Cratty, B. J., and Szczepanik, Sister M.: *The Effects of a Program of Learning Games Upon Selected Academic Abilities of Children with Learning Difficulties.* Washington, D.C., Bureau of Education for the Handicapped, Office of Education, 1971.
10. Dye, N. W. and Verz, P.S.: Growth changes in factorial structure by age and sex. *Genet Psychol Monogr. 78*:55–80, 1968.
11. Garrett, H. E.: A developmental theory of intelligence. *Am Psychol, 1*:372–378, 1946.
12. Kalm, S. B.: Development of mental abilities: An investigation of the differentiation hypothesis. *Can J Psychol, 32*:164–68, 1965.
13. Maccoby, Eleanor E., Dowley, E. M., and Hagen, J. W.: Activity level and intellectual functioning in normal pre-school children. *Child Dev, 36*:761–769, 1965.
14. Massari, D., Hayweiser, L., and Meyer, W. J.: Activity level and intellectual functioning in deprived pre-school children. *Dev Psychol, 1*:286–290, no. 33, 1969.

ENHANCING PERCEPTUAL MOTOR ABILITIES IN BLIND CHILDREN AND YOUTH*

∿∿

THERE ARE BASIC PHILOSOPHICAL and practical questions which arise, or should arise, when educational and recreational programs are designed for blind children. Should they be treated simply as children who cannot see, or are there basic perceptual, intellectual, and emotional differences to be considered in their makeup? For example, it is usually believed desirable to eliminate "blindisms" evidenced by congenitally blind children. These rocking movements and other rhythmic motoric behavior are used when the blind child engages in apparently pleasurable self-stimulation. To the sighted, however, this kind of behavior is unpleasant to observe; and, as it is usually felt that its continuance will impede the blind child socially, it is usually trained out of him. But what will replace it?

From scientific and semiscientific writings concerning these and other questions, various spurious assumptions have arisen during the past years. Some of these have been put to chase by research while others persist.

For example, the fabled obstacle sense of the blind has been reasonably well documented as having its genesis in reflected auditory cues. The more recent suggestion in popular magazines that there are certain blind people who can judge color through their finger tips is another example. The author had brief contact with this fable three years ago when asked to design a proposal

---

* Speech prepared for the California State Teachers of the Blind, Palo Alto, California, November, 12–13, 1971.

to determine whether the tactile perception of color was possible. A review of the literature on the manual perception of roughness and of heat brought the conclusion, prior to beginning the study, that the identification of colors through the finger tips was impossible. Fortunately the research was never consummated for it was learned at about the same time that the Russian woman who claimed to possess this magical power later admitted to looking under her blindfold!

Intelligent, congenitally blind children often possess abilities which are remarkably uneven in nature when compared to attributes evidenced by the sighted. For example, they frequently exhibit extensive vocabularies, but are not really sure of the nature of a traffic intersection. They may be able to read braille but have great difficulty signing their names in script. A study comparing a blind and a sighted child (pair of twins) recently completed in our laboratory revealed that, despite the blind girl's high intellect, she had only a vague concept of the human face, she could not throw or run accurately, and when asked to draw her favorite thing, could only inscribe a vague outline of her pet parakeet.[19]

Overall educational programs for blind children seem reasonably adequate during the middle years of childhood. Blind children enter school at about the age of five and learn braille as well as other traditional subjects. By the age of thirteen they can read and write braille adequately and usually graduate to junior high school to continue their studies.

The more marked deficiencies in the total educational program for blind children are in two areas, (a) pre-primary preparation for complexities of classroom learning, and (b) preparation which will enable the children to become mobile and self-sufficient in their environment during and after school years.

A review of the literature relating to data upon which these mobility training programs were established led to the conclusion that in most cases they employed techniques which were unsupported by objective evidence. The tendency for the blind to veer for example, while frequently observed, had not been measured. While investigators had studied the ability of rats to perceive gradient changes without vision, no effort had been made to evaluate this ability on the part of humans without sight.

It is with these considerations in mind that the research program was initiated. During the first year, basic normative data was obtained, and from this a mobility orientation test was constructed. This test measures an individual's ability to detect gradients and to walk straight without vision. Norms were compiled by assessing others similar in age. During the second year investigators attempted to ascertain the effects of brief practice upon various perceptual attributes. During the initial year of this investigation about 180 subjects were utilized, including forty-five children and youths from the ages of eight to nineteen. Also during the second year, fewer subjects were employed, but were detained for two days during which various tests were administered.

The following results were obtained when these data were analyzed:

1. The direction of a blind individual will veer, in the absence of auditory cues, is predictable and amounts to about 36° of angular rotation per 100 feet of forward progress, or about 1.25 inches of deviation per stride.

2. The blind are more sensitive to incline than to decline, or to left-right tilt in their walking surfaces.

3. Postural abnormalities, as evidenced by head torsion or tilt, and hand and leg dominance, as well as structural differences in leg length are not predictive of the direction nor of the amount of veer the blind will evidence.

4. Highly anxious blind individuals will walk significantly slower and will veer about twice as much while walking 100 feet as will the more relaxed blind person.

5. The blind will tend to be more sensitive to the slight curvature in pathways walked when it is opposite to the direction of their usual tendency to veer.

6. Congenitally blind adolescents will be more sensitive to gradients walked and will veer less than will the older adventitiously blinded. The former however, will frequently give evidence of a lack of left-right discrimination in their spatial field,

unlike the latter who have spent the majority of their lives with sight.

7. The longer an individual has been blind the less he will tend to veer, and the more accurately he can detect gradients.

8. The amount a blind individual will veer can be significantly reduced by permitting him to tactually inspect flexible wires indicating the amount and direction he veers.

9. The blind will usually overturn 90-degree turns and under-turn 180- and 360-degree turns when asked to do so in the absence of auditory cues. Training can correct this error by about 50 per cent.

10. A curb must have a radius of five feet before a blind individual can successfully detect its curvature, using the presently advocated cane techniques designed for this purpose.

It is believed that these findings may encourage mobility trainers to examine more closely some of their traditional practices, and will also tend to facilitate communication between the blind and the sighted by aiding each to better understand the reference system of the other. For example, it was found that while the sighted can easily detect horizontal deviations in the direction a blind individual is taking while attempting to walk a straight line, the blind are many times more sensitive to gradient changes than are the sighted who are visually inspecting the same surfaces. Similarly the curvature of curbs, which are obviously curved when the sighted inspect them, are difficult, if not impossible, for the blind to detect by employing the cane techniques presently advocated by mobility trainers.

While mobility trainers have at times placed heel lifts under the leg toward which the blind trainee veers, our findings suggest in several ways that the veering tendency is caused by some kind of perceptual distortion, rather than by structure. The blind, as well as the sighted, walk their legs, their legs do not walk them! A most interesting finding is that the direction to which an individual will habitually veer on the field can be predicted to a moderate degree by asking him to draw a straight line directly away from the center of his body while seated at a table.

Further evidence, which has important implications for the

perceptual-motor development and training of blind children, was gained when blind children were asked to walk through the curved twenty foot pathways with radii ranging from twelve to forty-two feet. Sixty per cent of the responses obtained from congenitally blind children were inaccurate, whereas the adventitiously blinded were usually correct in their judgments of these pathways. Although the congenitally blind were more accurate than the adventitiously blinded when walking straight and when judging gradients, one might conclude that the congenitally blind children did not have an accurate concept of laterality firmly established. Their ability to differentiate between left and right was extremely poor.

Most child development experts suggest that the child's basic perceptions of his body, including an awareness of its surfaces, as well as perception of the differences in the sides of the body, are formed early. By the age of six, it is usually suggested, the child's laterality as evidenced by hand-use is well established. It was apparent from our data that laterality was apparently not as well established in the congenitally blind.

These kinds of data suggest that in addition to an orderly presentation of increasingly complex objects for manual inspection, the congenitally blind child should be given training rather early in life designed to heighten his awareness of his body parts. Probably such training should accompany, and may enhance, the development of speech.

As soon as possible the infant should be made aware of his front and back, parts of his face and the location and name of his limbs. Furthermore, he should, in every possible way, be given tasks designed to enable him to understand various left-right concepts—that left and right directions change as he moves and that an individual facing him has a different left and right than he does. At the same time the child should be made to understand that his left arm and leg emerge from the left side of his body and he should be given tasks which enable him to locate himself relative to various objects. For example, using a box, various drills may be utilized which might help him to understand how to stand with his back, his front, his left side, and his right side nearest an object. If we are to believe the writings of Piaget regarding the importance of the sensory-tonic theory of perception advanced by Werner, it would seem that this kind of body image training is imperative for the child who has no opportunity to pair vision with movement.[14,18]

In a recent study on "The Body-Image of Blind Children," by Cratty and Sams,[8] 91 children were given a body-image survey form including verbal requests to identify planes of the body (front, back, and so forth) and body parts, in order to see the extent to which they had the potential to be taught and improve their body images. Accuracy was scored for responses to requests to make accurate movements of the body, to discriminate between left-right dimensions of the body, and to discriminate between the left and right of the tester. Analysis of the mean scores on the subtests suggested that body parts, body movements, and body planes were easiest and that directionality and laterality more difficult, with scores on the directionality section being significantly lower than scores on the laterality section, in which various left-right discriminations were required. Further analysis of the data suggested that (a) a score obtained by combining the subscores from the body-part and laterality sections was highly predictive of the total battery score; (b) though there were no sex differences, scores achieved by children with I.Q.s above 80, by the totally blind, and by older children were generally superior to scores achieved by children with I.Q.s of 79 and less, by the partially sighted, and by younger children under the age of twelve; (c) a moderate relationship was obtained between I.Q. and the total test battery score; and (d) though the total population was aware of body parts and the left-right discriminations required, they were totally incapable of projecting themselves into the tester's reference system (for example, naming another's left and right hand). On the basis of these findings, it was concluded that blind children's abilities to make accurate identifications of their body parts and to make other discriminations relative to the body image may be reliably assessed. The investigation also revealed significant intragroup differences and the relative order of difficulty, in the various subtests required, both differences having significant educational implications.

The study by Cratty and Sams argues that for the blind to gain any insight into the nature of space, they must be led through tasks that are carefully sequenced and accompanied by explicit instruction. Training sequences of this nature should be constructed. This conclusion was supported in a study by Walker.[17] Studying "The Effects of Training on the Body Image of Blind Children of Kindergarten Age," a training program consisting of individual daily lessons, each about fifteen minutes in length, was designed to increase knowledge of body parts, their relative positions, and their possibilities of movement in space. The sequences were largely based upon the sequences suggested by Cratty and Sams, with a fifteen-inch tall dissectable doll used as a teaching aid. The results of the study showed that a highly structured program of individualized training in body image is an effective means of increasing body image of kindergarten age blind children, and is a useful addition to the regular school program.

To further explore the educability of blind children in basic perceptual judgments, an eight-week training program was conducted from January to March, 1967 at the Frances Blend School in Los Angeles.[7] Thirty blind children from the ages of seven to fourteen years participated. It was hypothesized that practice in correcting veer and in facing movements would result in significant improvement in the ability of blind children to relocate their positions in space. The position relocation task consisted of attempting to reach a starting point after being led along the two legs of a right triangle. The hypotenuse was twenty-two feet. A group of control subjects matched according to age and I.Q. at the Foundation for the Junior Blind in Los Angeles were subjected to the same conditions before and after the test, but with no training given. Results of the study were most encouraging. For the children at Blend the average amount of veer at fifty feet before training was fifteen feet. After training the average veer was eight and one-half feet. This indicated a 42 per cent improvement after training. In relation to facing movement, the average error was again calculated. The average error for 90-degree turns before training was 22 degrees. After training this was reduced to 11 degrees. The average error for

180-degree turns before training was 42 degrees compared with an average error of 22 degrees after training. An overall improvement of approximately 50 per cent was demonstrated by the children in facing movement accuracy. Finally a mean error of twenty-six feet in position relocation was noted before training. The mean error after training was nineteen and one-half feet. This indicated a 24 per cent increase in performance. All of these training effects were statistically significant. Further analysis of the data, comparing the scores of the children under ten-years-old in the experimental group with those over ten-years-old resulted in the finding that both groups evidenced comparable improvement in the tasks they were trained for (correcting veer and facing movements) and in the task to which positive transfer was elicited (positive relocation).

More important than the statistical implications of this study are the practical ones. Responses from their teachers indicated that the blind child's concepts of left and right were enhanced through the training in facing movements. It was observed by the teachers that this improvement in laterality and directionality has not only physical but also intellectual implications. The academic curriculum in geography is an example, i.e. understanding longitude and latitude. After the experiment was completed, some of the children were also seen to walk to the training areas on their own and to engage in facing movement practice, correcting themselves by feeling the tapes with their toes. The positive results further reemphasize the importance of sound premobility programs in improving the blind child's basic perceptual judgments that assist his later mobility and orientation within the world.

Auditory training, as outlined in the research by Norton, can also be employed early in the life of the child.[12] Sounds can be paired with objects and with specific rooms in the home. At the same time sounds can be utilized to heighten the child's spatial orientation by placing them at various angles around him. Training of the obstacle sense, an awareness of the immediate presence of obstacles, would be a productive exercise for blind youth as they approach late childhood and early adolescence. A general awareness of obstacles through sound is relatively easy to gain, though a refinement of the obstacle sense may involve a more prolonged period of time during which more difficult discriminations must be made. A sequence of games could be played with the child to help train this sense. For example, the first stage of such a sequence of games could include putting up a cardboard square and having the child decide whether it is or is not there. The next stage could include having the child move in a circuitous pathway around several obstacles, walking through a "forest" without knocking down or touching "trees." As the child progresses, advanced games could be substituted by using obstacles of decreasing width or length. During the initial stages, the child might be encouraged to make noises, but as proficiency is acquired, he may be asked to depend only on noise produced from his footfalls or normal noise present in the situation. Other games could be played with obstacle shadows produced by sound. When a sound source is placed so that an obstacle is located between the perceiving individual and the noise, a shadow may be present which often enables the blind to perceive a reasonably accurate outline of the obstacle. Games, using this sound shadow, can be played with potentially helpful results. Cardboard obstacles could be placed side by side and as the child walks parallel to them, producing some kind of sound cue, he could be asked to estimate when gaps in these obstacles occur. More difficulty could be introduced by cutting small windows within single obstacles, and requiring the child to determine which of the obstacles he was passing contained such openings. As the blind child matures, he should be encouraged to attempt to guess when he is passing an open window, an open garage, or when the garage has a car in it. He should be confirmed or corrected immediately.

Good education begins first by establishing reasonable goals to be attained by students. Prior to instituting any program of education, two steps must be taken: (1) One must survey the extent to which the population to be educated possesses the attribute and/or the potential to learn the lesson taught; (2) study must then be carried out to determine the best ways to achieve expertise in the tasks in which proficiency is desired. The reason for a teacher's presence in the classroom is to change learners, whether it be tactile training, body image training, mobility education, or academic endeavors. Popham,[16] emphasizing the nature of change that occurs in learners, breaks the act of instruction down into categories which can be analyzed and subsequently improved for a better instructional method. Instrutional decision making (what to teach, how to teach, and procedures for evaluation of the teaching method) can be changed, and if done wisely, teaching behavior can be improved. Popham outlines a referenced instructional scheme to include (a) *objectives*—intended behavioral changes; (b) *preassessment*—measuring the learner to see how he stands in relation to the *objectives*, and if need be, to change the objectives so that they are more compatible with the learner; (c) *instruction*—the means of changing the learner; and (d) *evaluation*—assessing the quality of the instructional decision making, and if required, modifying it. When examining this behavior, empirical evidence must show that decisions are sound, hence the term "teacher empiricist" is used for an educator who follows this method. When working with the blind, decisions may have to be changed many times before the best workable solution is discovered, goals and methods being flexible in order to attain the most change.

It is thus believed that three basic improvements are needed in the educational programs for blind children: early, thorough, and systematic tactile training using objects of varying degrees of complexity; systematic body image training affording the blind child a better concept of his body, its location relative to objects, its parts, and its left-right dimensions; and a program of mobility education starting as soon as the child begins to walk. It is believed that through this three-pronged effort, and with a sound method of instruction, more blind children will arrive at schools emotionally prepared to participate in formal programs of education, and will emerge from school intellectually prepared to make meaningful contributions to themselves and to society.

BIBLIOGRAPHY

1. Burlingham, D.: Some notes on the development of the blind. *Psychoanal Study Child, 16*:121.
2. Carroll, Rev. Thomas J.: *Blindness*. Boston, Little, 1961.

3. Cratty, Bryant J.: *Human Behavior: Exploring Educational Processes.* Wolfe City, University Pr, 1971.
4. Cratty, Bryant J.: *Movement and Spatial Awareness in Blind Children and Youth.* Springfield, Thomas, 1971.
5. Cratty, Bryant J.: Perceptual thresholds of non-visual locomotion, Part I—the veering tendency, the perception of gradient, and of curvature in pathways: Inter-relationships, norms, inter-group comparison, and a mobility orientation test. Monograph, Department of Physical Education, University of California at Los Angeles, 1965.
6. Cratty, Bryant J., and Peterson, Carl: *The Educability of Blind Children in Spatial Orientations,* unpublished paper.
7. Cratty, Bryant J. and Sams, Theressa A.: *The Body-Image of Blind Children.* New York, American Foundation for the Blind, 1968, monograph.
8. Cratty, Bryant J. and Szczepanik, Sister Mark: *The Effects of a Program of Learning Games Upon Selected Academic Abilities in Children with Learning Difficulties.* 1970–1971, monograph sponsored jointly by the Joseph P. Kennedy Jr. Foundation, Washington, D.C., and the U.S. Department of Education's Bureau of Education for the Handicapped, University of California at Los Angeles, September, 1971.
9. Cratty, Bryant J. and Szczepanik, Sister Mark: *Sounds, Words, and Actions, 49 Movement Games to Enhance the Language Art Skills of Elementary School Children.* New York, Educational Activities, 1971.
10. Cratty, Bryant J. and Williams, Harriet G.: Perceptual thresholds of non-visual locomotion, Part II—the effects of brief practice upon veer, upon accuracy of facing movements, and upon position relocation: The perception of lateral tilt in pathways walked and of curvature of curbs; the relationship of accuracy of performance in selected table-top drawing tasks to the veering tendency and to position relocation. Monograph, Department of Physical Education, University of California at Los Angeles, 1966.
11. Norton, Fay-Tyler M.: Training hearing to greater usefulness. Manual, Cleveland Society for the Blind, 1960.
12. Parmalee, Arthur H. Jr.: Developmental studies of blind children: I. *The New Outlook for the Blind,* pp. 177–179, 1966.
13. Parmalee, H. A., and Fiske, C. E. and Wright, R. H.: The development of ten children with blindness as a result of retrolental fibroplasia, *AMA J Dis Child,* 98:198, 1959.
14. Piaget, Jean: *The Construction of Reality in the Child.* New York, Basic, 1954.
15. Popham, W. James: *The Teacher-Empiricist.* Los Angeles, Tinnon-Brown, 1970.
16. Shilling, C. W.: *Identification and Teaching of Auditory Cues for*

Traveling in the Blind, Groton, C. W. Shilling Auditory Research Center, 1963.

17. Walker, Don Lee: *The Effects of Training on the Body Image of Blind Children of Kindergarten Age.* A dissertation submitted in partial fulfillment of the requirements for the degree of Doctor of Education in the Department of Special Education of the Graduate School at George Peabody College for Teachers, August, 1971.

18. Werner, H. and Wapner, W.: Sensory-tonic field theory of perception. *J Pers, 18:*88–107, 1949.

19. Williams, Harriet G. and Beane, Virginia: A Comparison of Selected Behaviors of a Pair of Identical Twins, One Blind from Birth, unpublished paper.

20. Wolff, Peter: Developmental studies of blind children: II. *The New Outlook for the Blind,* June, vol. 64, 1966.

21. Cratty, Bryant J.: *Active Learning: Games to Enhance Academic Abilities.* Englewood Cliffs, P-H, 1971.

CHAPTER 15

PERCEPTUAL-MOTOR COMPETENCIES: EVALUATIVE TOOLS

Annotated Listing

EARLY DEVELOPMENTAL SCREENING includes scales appropriate for the severely brain damaged and the severely and profoundly retarded.

1. *The Gesell Scales* are often employed in this context, and contain scales appropriate for the identification of motor, as well as adaptative behaviors from the first months of life to the fourth and fifth years.

2. *The Vineland Scale of Social Competence*, contains seven sections, the first five of which are heavily loaded with motor items. The manual may be ordered from American Guidance Services Inc., Publishers Building, Circle Pines, Minnesota 55014.

3. *The Webb Scale* for evaluating the severely and profoundly retarded contains three subscales evaluating motor, sensory, and adaptative behaviors. It may be obtained from Dr. Ruth Webb, Glenwood State Hospital, Glenwood, Iowa.

4. *Fairview Social Skills Scale*, developed at Fairview State Hospital, Costa Mesa, California 92626, for the mildly and moderately retarded. It contains five subdivisions, including self-help skills, most of which are motor in nature. The author is Robert T. Ross, Fairview State Hospital.

5. *The Nihira Scale*, developed by Kazuo Nihira and his colleagues, with subscales for children and adults. This manual may

be ordered from The American Association on Mental Deficiency, 5201 Connecticut Ave. N.W., Washington, D.C. 20015.

6. *Denver Developmental Screening* contains four subscales including "gross motor" and "fine motor adaptive," a most helpful device, as it lists the percentage of children at various ages (1 month to 6 years) passing each of the many items under each subject heading. It may be ordered from Ladoca Project and Publishing Foundation Inc., East 51st Ave. and Lincoln St., Denver, Colorado, and was developed by Drs. William Frankenberg, and Josiah Dodds, University of Colorado School of Medicine.

Motor Ability Tests, appropriate for normals, and children suspected of having motor problems. Generally they require verbal comprehension on the part of the children tested.

1. *Cratty Scale,* a motor screening test, is appropriate for clinical use and has high reliability with trainable, educable, and NH populations. It includes six subscales, inadequate norms, averages from a population of middle class which children in the university elementary school UCLA, found in appendix of *Perceptual-Motor Behavior and Educational Processes,* Springfield, Illinois, Charles C Thomas, 1970. Norms (averages) also on trainables, educables. Ages four to twelve years of age.

2. *Oseretsky Test of Motor Proficiency,* American Guidance Service, Publishers Building, Circle Pines, Minnesota 55014. Pass-fail type tests ages four to fourteen years, need considerable equipment and time for administration.

3. *Purdue Perceptual-Motor Survey,* helpful as an observational tool, contains thirty items, in subscales including ocular pursuits, walking board tests, rhythmic writing, fitness, etc. It lacks precision of scoring as items are scored on a 1, 2, 3 and 4 point basis, may be insensitive to minor improvement in a pre post-test basis. Available from Charles E. Merrill Books, Columbus, Ohio.

4. *Frostig Movement Skills Test Battery,* developed by R. E. Orpet, termed as "experimental edition," contains twelve sub-

tests including tests of fine and gross coordination, muscle strength, balance, etc., twenty to twenty-five minutes for administration to a single child, forty-five minutes to three or four children, averages (inadequate norms) from six to twelve years of age. Published by Consulting Psychologists Press, 577 College Ave., Palo Alto, California 94306.

5. *The Fleishman Motor Ability and Fitness Scales.* Englewood Cliffs, New Jersey, Prentice-Hall, 1964. For ages twelve to eighteen, contains norms based upon 20,000 boys and girls, in all areas of motor ability, involving larger muscle groups.

PART IV

THE ATHLETE: PSYCHOLOGICAL CONSIDERATIONS

CHAPTER 16

PSYCHOLOGY OF THE SUPERIOR ATHLETE*

WHILE EARLY PHILOSOPHICAL WRITING concerning broad psychological questions appears in nineteenth century literature, scientific approaches to the study of the superior athlete, using the tools of the behavioral scientists, are primarily found in twentieth century writings. At the time of this writing, only a few scientists have even begun to explore this potentially useful, but extremely complex topic area.

At this point in time, I believe it is more correct to talk about the potential of psychological methodology in exploring the parameters which contribute to performance of the superior athlete, which suggests that a more appropriate title of this paper might be "Psychology *and* the Superior Athlete," rather than "Psychology *of* the Superior Athlete." An even more correct approach would be to use the plural term "athletes" rather than the singular, because most of the work carried out to date indicates that superior athletes not only appear in many different somatotypes, but that their psychological makeups also vary to a marked degree.

The interest in the psychology of superior athletes is widespread. For example, at the time of this writing the International Society for Psychology in Sport has a membership of about 1500. Several types of scholars in the countries of the world have focused their interest on the athlete, and at the same time, many routes have been taken to illuminate the interactions between athletic performance and various psychological variables. In some

---

* Speech to the Canadian Association of Sports Sciences, Quebec City, October 31, 1970.

countries there has been long-term interest focused upon athletes by psychologists, marked by fervor and dedication usually seen only in the political arena. In other countries a few psychologists or psychiatrists write in a leisurely way about the psychical states of athletes, with little data to support their often philosophical meanderings.

Within some countries (the United States is one), there are relatively few individuals devoting themselves to the study of superior athletes. In this same country a larger number are interested in studying various other aspects of motor activity, motor learning and motor development. In other countries, superior behavioral scientists, physiologists, and physicians are in close contact with the coaches of the national teams, and together their constant aim is to elicit better performances from the athletes representing their nations. In many of these latter nations, the study of the psychology of sport is often linked with the study of various aspects of bravery and courage which are important to efficient military performance, and also to studies of relationships of exercise and fitness to factory work.

This latter emphasis points to the fact that a study of the various factors impinging upon the superior athlete, and the manner in which the athlete overcomes adversity, also may disclose important information concerning how men and women meet life's stresses in a general way, not just within the sports arena.

As a younger man, I once or twice had speculated (fortunately never in writing) that I was somehow above or at least different from philosophers, who seemed to me at that time to pour out endless and not very important drivel. More recently, however, I have perhaps matured into the realization that one's philosophical viewpoint either covertly or overtly permeates most of what one does. It is usually best to consciously refer to a set of values prior to embarking on some type of scientific venture, while one is engaged in data collection, and also at the termination of a project.

With this framework in mind I would like to pose several questions to you concerning psychology of the superior athlete.

1) With whose primary welfare in mind should the psycholo-

gist carry out his duties? What if the poor mental health of the athlete actually contributes to his performance while at the same time detracting from his daily relationships with society, his family, and with himself? Should the psychologist attempt to rehabilitate the performer to the detriment of his performance, and perhaps the consternation of his coach? An associated question is, of course, "To whom is the psychologist responsible, his athlete-client or the total social subsystem in which the athlete resides?"

2) Should the psychologist be mainly concerned with eliciting maximum performance from a youth, or should he be more responsive to the long-term needs of the individual after his years of competition come to an end?

In addition to such moral questions there are others which the behavioral scientist should attempt to deal with when taking the time of athletes and coaches in the execution of research studies. For example:

1) If time is extended for studies of the athletes within a specific setting, just how valid will the findings be in helping both the athletes and coaches within the same setting? How much does the investigator intend to *give back* to those to whom he has obligated himself? Will the information be extended in a diplomatic manner and in a usable form?

2) Are the frequently encountered one-time studies of athletes, usually a restricted number within a specific setting, really worth carrying out? Can one really generalize from the findings of such studies? Most important, does a study of this nature represent a facet within a total program of research, or is it simply a device through which the psychologist is trying to solve an immediate problem facing him professionally? Or is the personal interest of the scientist only transitory and superficial?

The author does not have the answers to these queries, and is reminded of once reading that to appear wise one needs only to pose important questions!

Many readers are probably awaiting more specific answers to questions which concern those who are only beginning to become interested in the psychology of athletes, but whose primary interests lie elsewhere, i.e. in the physiological or medical parameters of athletic performance. Your questions are perhaps less philosophical, and more pointed. A scientist accustomed to finding a physiological-neurological mechanism underlying most of the behavior he studies, is perhaps already skeptical of anyone engaged in the study of perception or motivation in athletes. It is difficult, of course, to isolate the specific structures within the brain which mediate these rather diffuse human characteristics. Others are perhaps cognizant of the various neurological models which attempt to explain human learning; however anyone who is deeply enough into the literature should also be aware that these models are only somewhat poorly defined theories. They are not viable laws, such as the rather predictable principles which govern the transmission of nutrients through cell membranes, or which predict how the hydraulics within the cardio-vascular system operate in athletes and in nonathletes, as they engage in vigorous exercise.

Thus a brief summary of the more pertinent findings about superior athletes will be given in an attempt to outline some of the ways in which these findings were derived, and finally to illuminate some of the strategies employed by several clinical psychologists when attempting to apply these findings while working with superior athletes.

Much of the following information is contained in a book on which the author had the pleasure of collaborating with Dr. Miroslav Vanek.* He was the psychologist for the Czechoslovak-ian Olympic Team in 1968, and then went to Charles University in Prague.

The history of experimental studies in the psychology of sport began in the 1920's when laboratories in Russia were established. During the past fifty years, studies in Eastern Europe as well as in other parts of the globe have continued to explore various aspects of the subject. Some of the experimental strategies employed have included:

1) investigations of the type in which various performance tests conducted in laboratories and in the field predict athletic performance

---

* To be truthful, I acted as Dr. Vanek's transcriber and typist, while the primary content is from his research, clinical experiences, and theoretical postulations.

2) studies of the personal attributes which seem to be prevalent within a group of athletes engaged in specific sporting activity

3) studies of the perceptual as well as the motor attributes of athletes, and their relationship to superior performance

4) investigations of some of the social and psychological attributes within sports groups competing internationally

5) investigations of the manner in which the athlete may activate or deactivate himself prior to top-flight competition. Perhaps protocol used in these studies will be clearer upon reviewing some of the following slides.

The results of these and other investigations suggest that the following major findings are reasonably valid at the present time:

1) There appears to be no singularly identifiable athletic type of personality. Rather, the data available indicate that within specific events or types of events there are common types of personality traits found in groups of superior athletes. For example, there seems to be a common group of personality traits associated with events involving hard physical contact with others (wrestlers or linemen in American football), just as another complex of personality traits seems common to individuals engaging in the aesthetic events of free-exercise gymnastics and figure skating.

2) Based upon some emerging data, one is able to develop a general topology of sport activities based upon the type of stress inherent in the performance of each activity. Vanek has developed a five-category classification of sports, with subcategories including those in which injury or death are possible, those requiring total body coordination, those in which a single burst of power is important, those involving only hand-eye coordinations, and those in which one must anticipate the movements of (an)-other individual(s). It is obvious that several sports combine one or more of these classifications of attributes.

3) Athletes can be aided in improving performance by being exposed to techniques intended to either activate them or calm them down to the levels of arousal needed to perform their event in an optimal manner.

4) The reasons why superior athletes strive with the vigor they do are varied. To work well with a superior athlete, a clini-

cian must attempt to employ a variety of tools with which to assess his value system. Complicating the matter is the fact that a single value or group of values may at a given moment impinge upon the athlete's performance. A different value or group of values may, at another time, prompt him to perform well.

5) Acquainting athletes with the intellectual components of the events in which they are to participate should prove helpful. These cognitive elements may include knowledge of their unique psychological and physiological makeups; knowledge of the unique strategies and/or mechanics of the skills they are to master; as well as the potential social-cultural forces which are likely to impinge upon them prior to competition.

6) Potentially useful for coaches training athletic teams is an attempt to duplicate the psychological stresses, as far as possible in practice, which the same teams are likely to encounter in competition. These stresses may be introduced in the form of crowd noise, unusual or expected competitive situations as well as various "catch-up" or "hand-up" problems encountered by front-runners (or swimmers) or those holding back within individual racing competitions.

7) Assessing the potential of athletes through relatively simple and standard laboratory tests of various kinds, is not very helpful in predicting their performance under complex competitive conditions. Studies have shown that complex field tests similar to the sports abilities they must later evidence, are more helpful in this regard.

There are, of course, further problems in attempting to relate research findings of this type to the realities of sports competition. For example, the criterion a psychologist used to label his subjects "athletes" within his investigation, may not be the criterion used to select the individuals for a team competing for national honors. At the same time, the language used by the psychologist in explaining his findings, may prove difficult for some members of the coaching fraternity to interpret.

It is difficult to decipher why professional team members, upon whom millions of dollars are spent, and amateur teams competing within international competitions, do not have the benefit of consultation with a psychologist or psychiatrist when the unusual pressures to which they are subjected become too great to bear. Within the professional organization it would seem to be good business, while within the amateur Olympic ranks it not only would appear to be humane, but should also contribute to the superior performances usually desired by the country's inhabitants, who sponsor the teams with their tax dollars or out of their own pocketbooks. Yet in 1968 in Mexico City, only two psychologists were officially assigned to national teams, and one of these appeared only a few days before the competition, to test athletes the evening before each competed.*

Most important is the consensus that the most productive team of scientists within an athletic context consists of the triad of coach, physician (physiologist), and psychologist. It is hoped that this type of potentially fruitful model for action, in the years ahead, is seen to an increased degree within superior sports groups.

BIBLIOGRAPHY

1. Beisser, Arnold R.: *The Madness in Sports*. New York, Appleton, 1967.
2. Kenyon, Gerald (Ed.): *Proceedings of the Second International Congress for Sports Psychology*. Washington, D.C., Athletic Institute. Chicago, October, 1968.
3. Knapp, B.: *Skill in Sport*. London, Routledge & Kegan Paul, 1963.
4. Scott, Jack: *Athletics for Athletes*. Hayward, Quality Printing Service, 1969.
5. Vanek, Miroslav and Cratty, Bryant J.: *Psychology and the Superior Athlete*. London, Macmillan, 1970.

---

* One was Fredrich Blanz, a Finnish psychologist, the second was Professor Vanek who had worked continuously with the Czech team for three years prior to competition, accompanying them on two previous training expeditions to Mexico City's High Climate.

CHAPTER 17

CRITERIA FOR EVALUATING
SUPERIOR ATHLETES*

S INCE THE 1920's, in Eastern Europe, superior athletes have been exposed to various psychological measures. Despite the fact that the early beginnings of psychological measurements within an athletic context began about fifty years ago, at the time of this writing, there are relatively few sustained and sophisticated programs of psychological testing being carried out within the athletic context. The work that has been done, and is presently being carried out, is marked by the inclusion of measures of questionable validity, is seen in programs which are not sustained over periods of time, and has often been supervised by individuals who are somewhat less than competent.

The psychological research dealing with the many factors which might impinge upon superior athletic performance is somewhat scattered throughout the world, is often marked by "one-short" efforts which are not sustained over a period of time, and is characterized by research designs, sampling techniques, and data treatment procedures which are *often less than adequate.*

Despite this somewhat less than optimistic evaluation of current assessment practices, there are helpful guidelines contained within the literature which suggest sound principles upon which valid and helpful evaluation programs might be based. It shall be the purpose here to attempt to illuminate some of these principles.

---

* Prepared for the 1st International Symposium on Art and Science of Coaching, in Toronto, Canada, October 1st to 5th, 1971: sponsored by the Coaching Association of Canada, the Canadian Olympic Association and the Fitness Institute of Ontario, Canada.

Conceived of broadly, the psychological assessment of athletes should probably include measures of three rather global dimensions of personality and performance. These include (a) the assessment of physical performances of various kinds, including psychomotor measures, fitness and strength tests, and the like; (2) the measurement of rather stable personality traits; and (3) the evaluation of more dynamic components of the personality, including temporary motivational states, transitory anxiety levels, and the like.

The information obtained from a thorough and well conceived program of evaluation may also be employed in three ways: (a) for the purposes of basic research, to discover reasonably valid principles through which to understand athletic performance, the functioning of men and women under stress, and possibly to understand how to encourage more superior performance in athletes; (b) to permit the athlete to gain a better understanding of himself, of his interactions with other people and with conditions within the athletic context; and (c) to enable the coach, and others who are attempting to assist him, to understand the athlete better, and to direct his efforts more efficiently, accompanied by more satisfactory interpersonal communication.

The discussion which follows will attempt to cover several aspects of a program of psychological assessment of athletes; including operational considerations concerning the frequency of testing periods, as well as the qualifications of personnel administering and interpreting the tests. Additional suggestions concerning the content of testing programs will be included. The essay concludes by enumerating some of the philosophical and ethical considerations which should accompany a program of psychological assessment.

Components of a Psychological Assessment Program

As was mentioned above there are at least three types of assessment instruments which might be employed when evaluating the potential, general psychological makeup of athletes: those assessing physical capacities, instruments designed to sample rather basic and stable personality traits, and those intended to evaluate more transitory qualities in the athlete. The thorough evaluation of basic, physical ability attributes, is probably more desirable when attempting to assess the potentials in a group of novices than when evaluating the superior athlete, already demonstrating his or her ability to compete in world-class competitions.

Such basic ability measures as outlined by Fleishman, and others, however, when applied to superior athletes, might reveal which ones seem to be exerting an undue amount of motivation to compensate for possible basic physical ability deficiencies. While on the other hand, this type of basic psychomotor assessment might also identify athletes who possess superior physical qualities, and yet who do not seem to work up to their potential.

At the same time, to subject world-class athletes to basic psychomotor tests and to evaluations of their basic motor capacities would seem superfluous in so far as they are already demonstrating superior performance at the sport in which they are engaged. In Eastern Europe it has been the practice to confront athletes with laboratory and field tests reflecting motor abilities; and yet at the same time the researchers and clinicians who have employed these measures have found that unless the laboratory and/or field test almost exactly duplicates the sport in which the athlete is evidencing proficiency, there is little predictive value to be gained by inspecting the performance scores in the former.

PERSONALITY TRAIT MEASURES. A favorite type of measure employed by sports psychologists throughout the world has been the personality test. At times, groups of athletes within a given performance group have been surveyed, and profiles drawn upon which to compare the test scores of a single athlete. At other times, the information obtained from such tests when surveyed by the athlete himself, has aided him to gain a better understanding of the dimensions of his behavior. In still other instances the results of such testing have been surveyed by the coach and team physician, and compared to the athlete's daily, weekly, and yearly performances. Sometimes the athlete is fully oriented as to the pusposes of the testing program to which he is to be subjected, while at other times he is not.

In general, it is believed that the following criteria should be considered when administering and evaluating the results of personality tests which may be administered to superior world-class athletes:

1. The testing program should be fully explained, and the results of the testing should be clearly evaluated following the collection of personality test data. If full cooperation is to be expected, sophisticated athletes should not be kept in the dark about the purposes of the testing, the rationale underlying the test to which they are exposed, or the short-comings of such tests.

2. The kind of thorough orientation and evaluation outlined in 1 above, necessitates that personality tests be administered by those qualified in their use and interpretation, that is, a qualified psychologist. Mail-order psychological evaluations administered by a coach, and sent elsewhere for interpretation, simply do not fulfill either adequate moral or scientific conditions which should surround the collection of relatively sensitive personal information and feelings of human beings.

3. The personality tests employed should be suitable for administration to individuals who are reasonably healthy psychologically. The Minnesota Multiphasic Personality Inventory, often employed to assess athletes, for example, is in truth designed to screen large populations of individuals for the possible presence of rather severe psychiatric problems, and is not suited for evaluating the personality parameters of a reasonably normal population.

4. The tests administered should be scientifically valid and reliable. Their validity should be ascertained by the individual conducting the test, by reviewing the literature presented to support them and by the social scientist constructing the test. Such tests should be valid from a factor analytic standpoint, that is, each dimension measured by the test should be unique unto itself and not overlap other factors; additionally the factors identified by the test should be relatively stable over time, and verifiable through the clinical assessment of the individuals taking the test and through the administration of other tests purporting to evaluate the same qualities.

Because of its easy administration and the fact that it has been translated into several languages the Cattell 16 PF questionnaire has been employed often. However, many questions arise as to whether there are as many as sixteen separate and stable personality dimensions, rather than six or eight. Moreover, in a review in Buros' Mental Measurement Yearbook, it was stated that the primary use of the Cattell should be in basic research, rather than in clinical assessment upon which personal counseling decisions may be based.

A recent contribution which may provide a helpful alternate to the Cattell 16 PF, is the Comrey Personality Scale, a device which has undergone over fifteen years of refinement and seems valid based upon factor analyses which have taken into consideration when to stop rotating factors, and what communalities to use. This scale results in the identification of eight dimensions of personality, and is of potential use to the sports psychologist attempting to obtain data relative to rather stable personality dimensions of the athletes with whom he is dealing.*

5. More than one measure of important personality characteristics, i.e. anxiety, should be undertaken to ascertain whether indeed the score obtained might have been an artifact of a specific test administered.

6. Reasonably frequent administrations of a given personality test may be undertaken, perhaps using several forms of the test, to ascertain the manner in which certain trait scores recorded may be transitory vs. stable. This rather frequent administration might prove to be particularly helpful if carried out well before, as well as just prior to competition.

7. Despite the advice given in 6, above, caution should be exercised so that the time taken to administer personality tests is not so prolonged that it feels oppressive to the athletes concerned. Hostility, lack of cooperation, and similar symptoms will necessarily corrupt personality trait measures, and reflect too fre-

---

* These dimensions include trust vs. defensiveness, orderliness vs. lack of compulsion, social conformity vs. rebelliousness, activity vs. lack of energy, emotional stability vs. neuroticism, extraversion vs. introversion, masculinity vs. femininity, and empathy vs. egocentricism.

quent and too expansive testing programs administered by enterprising sports psychologists.

8. Testing programs involving personality tests should be taken by coaches as well as by the athletes. With this approach, the athletes and coaches may then, with the help of their psychologist, discover the possible reasons underlying interpersonal communication problems which may beset them.

9. Care should be taken to make respondents understand the limitations of personality tests; and at the same time personality test data should be considered within the total context comprising other information obtained from the respondents. For example, obtaining a detailed autobiography from athletes often aids in the interpretation of their personality trait scores, as well as aiding the coach and psychologist to determine the transitory vs. stable nature of the personality scores obtained.

10. Personality scores obtained often lead toward the interpretation of other measures obtained. For example, a sociogram identifying social isolates on a team, together with trait scores evidencing lack of sociability and/or introversion, suggests that the athlete may be relatively comfortable with the social isolation in which he finds himself. On the other hand, personality trait scores evidencing high need for approval by others, together with data indicating lack of social acceptance by other team members combine to present a different picture of the possible feelings an athlete may harbor relative to the social isolation he may be experiencing.

In summary, it is suggested that personality tests be employed primarily to help an athlete understand himself, and to improve his communication with his coach. At the same time valid and reliable personality tests should be carefully interpreted before and after their administration to all concerned. At the same time it should be clearly understood by the respondents just how such data will be employed after it is collected. And finally, personality trait scores should be interpreted within a total program of evaluation including sociological data, biographical information, measurements of performance capacities, and the more transitory and situational measures of mood and temperament which will be discussed briefly below.

Measure of Dynamic Personality States

Many of the psychological reasons * an individual performs well, or poorly, are dependent not only upon relatively stable measures of personality, but also upon more temporary mood states. For example, the literature documents the existence in people of a rather stable measure of what might be termed general or trait anxiety, versus what has been termed situational anxiety.

Even though an individual may be described as generally being motivated by one or more things important to him, at any given moment in time the degree of importance the performer may attach to some kind of specific motivational condition may vary markedly from the value he places upon the same condition at another moment in time.

Those constructing paper and pencil measures of personality, attitude, temperament, and motivation have long recognized the transitory nature of at least a part of the scores obtained from such measures. The sport psychologist should also recognize this rather unstable portion of the personality which may vary from moment to moment, particularly when the individual faces the emotionally taxing prospect of exhibiting his physical skills within highly competitive circumstances.

To tap the nature of these rather transitional mood states the psychologist may engage in several strategies.

1. Rather short measures of personality, anxiety and similar qualities may be employed frequently within the training regime, particularly as the day of the contest nears.

2. The psychologist should become familiar with measures specifically designed to evaluate temporary motivational states. Cattell's Motivational Analysis Test is an example of this type of measure, containing sections evaluating fear attitudes, sentiment to career, feelings about self, and similar dynamic qualities within the total personality structure.

---

* It is apparent that the primary reasons an individual performs well or poorly are dependent upon the physical abilities he brings with him to the performance situation. At the same time determining the per cent of his performance dependent upon temporary and stable moods and traits, vs. the per cent governed by his physical abilities is a most difficult undertaking.

Cattell and others have pointed out several reasons why individuals evidence changes in these kinds of transitory or surface traits, including the fact that individuals tend to mold the personal tendencies of those who seem to be, or who seem to move, too far from some kind of average. This tendency for a group to engage in coercion to some biosocial mean, is present in an athletic team, as well as within a more global section of society. Thus, with increased exposure to a team setting, these kinds of semipermanent characteristics may emerge and fluctuate from time to time. The changes in the personality traits of young age group swimmers, noted over a period of time by Bruce Ogilvie [9] and Thomas Tutko, may be one example of the team's social context molding the surface personality traits of team members.

Summary

Within these few pages it has been possible to offer only a few superficial guidelines for the evaluation of superior athletes. Most important is the realization on the part of the psychologist that professionally sound and ethical testing and counseling procedures should be exercised within the potentially stressful athletic context, with perhaps even more care than is done in other kinds of occupational, or educational environments.

Valid tests should be employed, and rather than relying upon the results of a single test when counseling athletes, a number of measures should be obtained. Direct questionnaires concerning mood state and biographical data together with more obtuse measures of personality should be used to compliment each other.

Care should be taken not to offend the athlete's intelligence, nor to upset his psychological well-being when embarking upon an evaluation program, and when interpreting the results at its completion. And finally, the results of such a testing program are of more use in the counseling of individual athletes than in formulating preconceived notions of what a typical athlete in a given sport must conform to, relative to his physical performance and stable and surface personality trait measures.

BIBLIOGRAPHY

1. Cattell, Raymond B.: *The Scientific Analysis of Personality*. Baltimore, Penguin, 1965.
2. Comrey, Andrew L.: Comrey Personality Scales. San Diego, California: Educational and Industrial Testing Service, 1971.
3. Cratty, Bryant J.: Anxiety, stress, and tension. In Cratty, Bryant J.: *Movement Behavior and Motor Learning*, 2nd ed. Philadelphia, Lea & Febiger, 1967.
4. Hathaway, H. and McKinley, B.: *Minnesota Multiphasic Personality Inventory*. New York, The Psychological Corporation, 1943.
5. Ikegami, Kinji: Character and personality changes in the athlete. In Kenyon, Gerald S. (Ed.): *Contemporary Psychology of Sport*. Chicago, Athletic Institute, 1970.
6. Kane, John E.: Personality and physical abilities. In Kenyon, Gerald S. (Ed.): *Contemporary Psychology of Sports*. Chicago, Athletic Institute, 1970.
7. Malumphy, Theresa M.: *The Assessment of Personality and General Background of Women Participating in Regional and National Inter-collegiate Competition*, an unpublished monograph partially supported by the University of Oregon Graduate School.
8. Maslow, Abraham H.: *Motivation and Personality*, 2nd ed. New York, Har-Row, 1970.
9. Ogilvie, Bruce C.: Psychological consistencies within the personality. *JAMA*, Special Olympic year edition, September–October, 1968.
10. Rushall, Brent S.: An evaluation of the relationship between personality and physical performance categories. In Kenyon, Gerald S. (Ed.): *Contemporary Psychology of Sport*. Chicago, Athletic Institute, 1970.
11. Rushall, Brent S.: Some practical applications of personality information to athletics. In Kenyon, Gerald S. (Ed.): *Contemporary Psychology of Sport*. Chicago, Athletic Institute, 1970.
12. Vanek, Miroslav and Cratty, Bryant J.: The evaluation of the superior athlete. In Vanek, Miroslav and Cratty, Bryant J.: *Psychology and the Superior Athlete*. Toronto, Macmillan, 1970.
13. Vanek, Miroslav and Hosek, V.: Methodological problems in psychodiagnostic investigations of the personality of sportsmen. In Kenyon, Gerald S. (Ed.): *Contemporary Psychology of Sport*. Chicago, Athletic Institute, 1970.

CURRENT RESEARCH AND PRINCIPLES

OF LEARNING AND TRANSFER OF

INTEREST TO THE COACH*

INCREASINGLY, behavioral scientists are studying the athlete and
his performance in order to understand better the contribution of motor activity to the human personality. This is evident in
the formation of several international societies for the study of
psychological and sociological variables important to the understanding of sports participation and of the sportsmen themselves.
In 1965, the First International Congress of the Psychology of
Sport met. Over two hundred educators, psychiatrists, and physical educators presented papers and engaged in discussions about
common interests.

Since then, the North American Society for Psychology in
Sport and Physical Activity was formed and a Second International Congress was held in October, 1968 in Washington, D.C.
A committee on sports sociology, a division of the International
Council for Sport and Physical Education, has met several times,
culminating in an International Seminar held in Cologne, Ger-
many during April, 1966, with the theme "Small Group Research
in Sport" and the publication of the *International Review of
Sport Sociology*.

Publications have appeared in the English language within
recent years dealing with the personality of the athlete,[2,19] the

* Prepared for the 1st International Symposium on Art and Science of Coaching,
in Toronto, Canada, October 1st to the 5th, 1971; sponsored by the Coaching
Association of Canada, the Canadian Olympic Association, and the Fitness Institute of Ontario, Canada.

nature of sport in society, the influence of sport on society and on the individual,[5] and containing detailed discussions of various psychological parameters of motor behavior.[4,6,14] Motivation in games has been discussed in a text written by fifty-six psychiatrists and psychologists.[15]

Foreign texts have also appeared dealing with similar topics. Ferrucio Antonelli,[1] for example, has written a book based upon the results of psychoanalysis of more than 200 Italian athletes. The Russian scientists have also been active writers about motor behavior.[21]

While some of these literary efforts have merely echoed the familiar cliches concerning the influence of sport upon the human personality, others have presented exact data which may dispel some of the folklore connected with sports activity which in the past has often been accepted with something approaching evangelical intensity. The positive value of sport in personality development has been questioned by some,[2] while others argue that the role of teamwork in the production of winning effort should be closely examined.[5,10,11]

Athletes and coaches are becoming more sophisticated when subjected to the outpourings of individuals championing some new training system. Some are beginning to ask for data which underlie statements supposedly supporting the place of physical education and athletics in the educational program. The result of this questioning has been an increased number of research studies to which practitioners have varying degrees of access.

Interpreting the implications derived from recent research presents several problems. For example, not all research in motor activity has any immediate practical significance. Research with the National Science Foundation dealing with figural aftereffects has very few implications for practice, except for the suggestion that swinging two bats prior to using a single one probably does not help very much.[7] Not all practice in physical education programs needs to be verified or substantiated by a research study.

When interpreting the practical facets of research, the question enters: Just what is important to whom? Most research studies in the behavioral sciences dealing with perception, motivation, personality, learning, and social psychology might have relevance to the complex personal and social interactions occurring within a single hour in a physical education class.

A definition of new research might also require interpretation. Most of the research produced within the last thirty years relevant to motor learning, transfer of training and similar subjects is ignored by the majority of coaches and physical educators when planning their day's lessons. Physical educators still conduct vigorous exercise programs at the beginning of class periods, so that their students are too tired to learn effectively; the pregame meal still consists of hard to digest low-energy steak; and many drills conducted in practice sessions are certain to produce negative transfer to the game.

Determining what is truth poses formidable problems. Must a finding be echoed in numerous research studies or will a single investigation's findings suffice when attempting to establish the truth? What is the truth when conflicting findings are available? And what are criteria for determining good research?

Despite the problems discussed in the preceding paragraphs, the following is an attempt to outline some findings related to the teaching of sports skills in physical education and athletics in which research has given us some tentative answers. Some of these findings stem from research laboratories of psychologists, while others are found in literature produced by physical educators, social psychologists and educators.

What Transfers?

Most teaching is teaching for transfer. The attempt is to devise drills which will transfer to the total game situation. Skills taught on Monday, it is hoped, will transfer to those complex ones taught on Wednesday. And yet well-established principles are often ignored when teaching physical education. Some "tip-in" drills in basketball seem certain to teach the players not to tip the ball in the hoop when game time arrives. Defensive backs are taught to cross their feet when moving sideways down the field during practice, while the extent to which this occurs in a game is closely related to how often the opposition scores.[9]

Transfer will occur to the extent to which a lead-up drill contains responses or response elements similar to those in the total game skill they purport to enhance. While there is a tendency to learn agility drills (to acquire certain response sets), in general the drills must be specifically related to the complex skill they propose to help.

Transfer of training will be effective to the extent to which cognitive bridges are built between the two skills. Children should be informed why they are performing various lead-up drills or games, rather than simply being pushed through exercises which may be meaningless to them.

Transfer will occur to the extent that a number of response patterns inherent to the final reference task are practiced. Learning how to perform many variations of a single skill is more helpful than prolonged practice on only one of several possible modifications of the task.

Mental Practice

Improvement can be gained in motor skills by merely thinking about them. Usually it is found that some optimum combination of motor and mental practice will facilitate the teaching and learning of a motor skill. Children in classes should be urged to think through the activity prior to performing it and to spend time watching and thinking about others' actions when they are in close proximity.

We Can Often Learn Best When No Practice Is Engaged In!

There are from 400 to 500 studies concerned with the influence of the timing of practice schedules upon the learning of mental and motor tasks.[4] Much of this work indicates that physical educators are usually prone to mass practice, to the detriment of the skill to be learned. A student once had this principle vividly portrayed to her when she found that a no-practice control group improved more in volleyball service skill than did two other groups who were given visual demonstration and verbal rehearsal of the skill over a three-day period.

Generally it is probably best to initially mass practice, and then as boredom and psychological fatigue begin to blunt the performance curve, practice should be spaced. This, of course, can be accomplished independent of the number of times physical education is taught per week, as numerous skills may be practiced, or not practiced, within a single week or within a single period.

The Factors in Learning

Several studies from the laboratories of the psychologists have attempted to determine what factors are important during various stages within the learning process.[12] Generally, with regard to motor skills, it is concluded that nonmotor factors, including spatiality, knowledge of mechanical principles and the like, are more important during the initial stages of learning, while during the final stages, the motor factors, such as movement, speed, reaction time and the like, become more influential. These findings have been followed up by studies in which the investigators have geared their instructions to the manner in which various factors will emerge, emphasizing, for example, "move fast" just before movement speed becomes an important variable in the performance of the task.[12]

The Effects of Close Affiliation Among Team Members

The causes for positive and negative group effort in athletic competitions are subtle and varied.[5] An examination of the literature in the psychology of small, group interaction reveals that the interaction of two primary types of motives is of paramount importance when attempting to elicit maximum group effort. One of these motives involves the need to achieve optimum performance, while the second is the need for affiliation, which may be met to varying degrees by membership in a group.

It is usually assumed that these two needs are complementary, that the "we" feeling of a group promotes greater group effort; and conversely, heightened group effort enhances close feelings among group members. There are several studies, however, which indicate that these two feelings on the part of team members may at times be in opposition to one another.[8,10] If individuals are on a team primarily to meet personal needs for affiliation, the total group performance may suffer. For example, in one study completed by the author, it was found that when two groups were brought together to engage separately in a unique, gross motor task (such as maze running while blindfolded), a closely knit fraternity group who had previously been associated in social activities performed more poorly than did a group whose members had not met previous to the experiment.[8] These findings were contrary to the hypothesis, for it had been reasoned that the fraternity group (the primary group), with established lines of communication and leaders previously established, would perform better.

A search for the reason for the findings was fruitful. It was found that the tendency of the previously affiliated group was to engage in social chatter instead of fruitful interactions between the trials allotted to them; whereas the members of the secondary group, who had had no previous affiliation, performed better since no social noise interfered with their attempts to solve the task's complexities. Instead this latter group confined its discussions to the problem at hand, that is, how to hold one's hand on the pathway's railing, the nature of the pattern they were attempting to traverse, and similar subproblems.

The previously established social leaders of the primary group were ineffective in leading their groups in the motor problem that they were confronted with; whereas the leaders of the secondary groups were selected by the group members for their competency at the task at hand after they had determined who had run the maze in the fastest time.

It is obvious that sports teams whose members are constantly in conflict with one another will not perform well, for among other things they will dissipate much of the leadership energy of the group and the disruption of helpful group interactions may also result in poor effort in the game itself. On the other hand, it is equally obvious upon consulting the research cited as well as earlier studies by Fiedler[10] and others that the amount of group effort directed toward the task at hand may be dissipated if the group is socially too close to one another.

These findings pose special problems for coaches of athletic teams, for it is equally true that individuals will tend to affiliate socially if continually in close physical proximity.[19] Friendships will develop to a great extent if this affiliation has resulted in mutual success (winning games).[25] Thus the effective coach should recognize that for optimum group effort the group members must be primarily focused upon successful performance for its own sake, rather than upon the need for affiliation. A winning team may begin to lose games because of the heightened mutual attractiveness of individuals in the group as a result of their initial winning efforts.

A coach should not become particularly disturbed if at times interpersonal tensions, particularly between the better performing members and those who are perceived to inhibit group effort, are evidenced on athletic teams. This hostility may in reality be a healthy thing, for the individual showing displeasure is making it quite apparent that he values winning more than he does the friendship of his poorer performing teammates. At the same time it should be the coach's attempt to produce an optimum amount of "group-win" tension, while engendering an optimum amount of "we" feeling between team members. If these two conditions are met, the best team performance should be forthcoming.

Essentially there is little literature dealing with learning and transfer of training, and with the social psychology of human interactions which does not hold implications upon the athletic environment. The material outlined above is meant only to arouse the interest of the reader, which will hopefully lead to a more thorough pursuit of the available material, some of which is listed in the following bibliography.

BIBLIOGRAPHY

1. Antonelli, Ferrucio: *Psicologia e Psicopatologia dello Sport.* Rome, Leonardo Edizioni Scientifiche, 1963.
2. Beisser, Arnold R.: *The Madness in Sports: Psychosocial Observations on Sports.* New York, Appleton, 1967.
3. Cratty, Bryant J.: *Human Behavior: Exploring Educational Processes,* 1st ed. Wolfe City, University Pr, 1971.
4. Cratty, Bryant J.: *Movement Behavior and Motor Learning,* 2nd ed. Philadelphia, Lea & Febiger, 1967.
5. Cratty, Bryant J.: *Social Dimensions of Physical Activity.* Englewood Cliffs, P-H, 1967.
6. Cratty, Bryant J.: *Psychology and Physical Activity.* Englewood Cliffs, P-H, 1968.
7. Cratty, Bryant J. and Duffy, Kirt E.: *Relationships Between Figural After-Effects Elicited by Selected Bodily Movements.* Part I, National Science Foundation Grant Number NSF GB 5664, August, 1967.

8. Cratty, Bryant J. and Sage, Jack N.: The effects of primary and secondary group interaction upon improvement in a complex movement task. *Res Q, 35:*265–274, 1964.
9. Ellis, Henry: *The Transfer of Learning.* New York, Macmillan, 1965.
10. Fiedler, F. E.: Assumed similarity measures as predictors of team effectiveness. *J. Abnorm. Soc. Psychol.,* 49, 381–388, 1954.
11. Fiedler, F. E., Washington, W. G., and Blaisdell, F. G., "Unconscious Attitudes as Correlates of Sociometric Choice in a Social Group," *J Abnorm Soc Psychol,* 47:790–796, 1952.
12. Fleishman, Edwin A.: A relationship between incentive motivation and ability level in psychomotor performance. *J Exp Psychol, 56:*78–81, 1958.
13. French, Elizabeth G.: Motivation as a variable in work partner selection. *J Abnorm Soc Psychol, 51:*96–99, 1956.
14. Knapp, Barbara: *Skill in Sport: The Attainment of Proficiency.* New Rochelle, Sportshelf, 1963.
15. Knight, James and Slovenko, Ralph: *Motivations in Play, Games, and Sports.* Springfield, Thomas, 1967.
16. Lavery, J. J.: The effect of one-trial delay in knowledge of results on the acquisition and retention of a tossing skill. *Am J Psychol,* 77:437–443, 1964.
17. Myers, A.: Team competition, success, and the adjustment of group members. *J Abnorm Soc Psychol,* 65:325–332, 1962.
18. Nelson, Dale O.: Leadership in sports. *Res Q, 37:*268–275, 1966.
19. Ogilvie, Bruce C., and Tutko, Thomas A.: *Problem Athletes and How to Handle Them.* London, Pelham Books, Ltd., 1966.
20. Pepiton, A. and Kleiner, R.: The effects of threat and frustration on group cohesiveness. *J Abnorm Soc Psychol, 54:*192–199, 1957.
21. Rudik, P. A. and Puni, A. T. (Eds.): *Psychological Training of the Sportsman.* Moscow, Russia (USSR), Academy of Education of the Russian Federation, 1965.
22. Sage, George H.: *Introduction to Motor-Behavior: A Neuropsychological Approach.* Reading, A-W, 1971.
23. Sherif, M. and Sherif, Carolyn: *Groups in Harmony and Tension.* New York: Har-Row, 1953.
24. Smith, Leon E. (Ed.): *Psychology of Motor Learning.* Chicago, The Athletic Institute, 1970.
25. Wilson, Warner and Miller, Norman: Shifts in evaluations of participants following inter-group competition. *J Abnorm Soc Psychol,* 63:428–431, 1961.
26. Ziegarnik, Bluma: Uber das Behalten von erledigten und unerledigten Handlugen. *Psychol Forsch,* 9:1–85, 1927.
27. Vanek, Miroslav and Cratty, Bryant J.: *Psychology and the Superior Athlete.* New York, Macmillan, 1970.

CHAPTER 19

PSYCHOLOGICAL HEALTH IN ATHLETICS: MODELS FOR MAINTENANCE

S ELDOM A WEEK PASSES without an item in the sports pages of our newspapers being devoted to some aspect or outcome of an emotional problem evidenced by a professional athlete. Indeed one could gain the impression that our cadres of professional competitors are overrun with psychological cripples. And while the incidence is not as high as might be gained from a perusal of the headlines, professional athletes performing under the glare of publicity, in situations in which success and failure are easily measurable, do have their problems. For example, a professional athlete recently told me that from five to seven young athletes in a forty-man team are likely to evidence symptoms of stomach ulcers during a single season, while symptoms of minor and major emotional disturbances may be seen in a third to a half of all competitors during a sport season, depending upon the sport and the length of the season.

Emotional problems among athletic groups are not only found in the professional ranks. It has been estimated that within a forty- to sixty-member roster of a high school football team, one or two are on the verge of a nervous breakdown during a season, while at least twelve to fifteen others could benefit from some kind of psychiatric or psychological counseling, due to the stresses imposed by their sport. The high school athlete is often too immature to bear the whole brunt of competition, impacts often unaccompanied by support from an adult figure close to him. Indeed the youngster may be derided daily by his coach, periodically by the press, and may even be rejected by members of his family, if the team is not having a successful season. This combination of forces can prove overwhelming, and even culminate in suicide as occurred recently in the northwestern part of the United States. Athletics for the maturing boy is often a wholesome method of self-expression, an uplifting part of his life, and one which provides him with important evidence of self-realization. At the same time athletic success, and team membership, is often the glue which is holding a youngster together—a boy or girl whose family and other psychosocial conditions may be less than supportive, or stable. If this glue evaporates when the boy is denied team membership or achieves less than expected success, his entire personality may evidence a concomitant disintegration with accompanying symptoms of unrest, despair or even inappropriate aggression and asocial behaviors.

Even the apparently stable productive athlete, in the high school, in preadolescent sport or professional ranks, may undergo emotional changes as he competes for several years or more which will result in psychological trauma. Arnold Beisser has described well some of the problems encountered by athletes at career's end.[1] The loss of a way of expressing one's aggressions as the season or career terminates may result in severe adjustment problems; the loss of status and self-respect felt by high school and college athletes, as their talents do not permit them to ascend to the next higher level of competition may similarly cause them to need professional help in the realignment of values, energies and general outlook upon life. Career's end may come following the finish of a Little League career when the boy or girl finds he or she cannot make the high school team, when the high school star finds that his talents are not desired by college or university coaches, when the professional athlete finds himself with a crippling injury, or when the symptoms of aging prove debilitating.

Emotional upset has also been superficially studied in Little League competition. Vera Skubic, for example, found via questionnaires that about one third of all the young (pre-high school) competitors in baseball evidenced various kinds of signs indicating undue emotional unrest. These included difficulty in eating, unrest at night and similar symptoms. It is interesting to note that in this study it was found that these symptoms appeared more often among children who were winning, than among losers.

It is fair to point out that other investigators have suggested that in general the college or grade school athlete is rated as more emotionally healthy than noncompetitors. At the same time the data forming the bases of these speculations are generally inferential rather than the result of careful research, in which athletes and nonathletes are carefully compared, keeping constant such factors as I.Q., academic achievement, age and sex.

Despite the evidence that there tend to be rather marked emotional problems among athletic groups at all levels, there have been few organized attempts by athletic organizations and individuals in this country pointed toward the illumination and correction of these conditions. In contrast, there is, at the time of this writing, an effort underway to provide a central research and service effort directed toward the study and remediation of physical injuries in athletes, organized primarily by those interested in sports medicine.

However, as most agree, athletic endeavor is an emotional as well as a physical undertaking; it is inconceivable to this writer why large and expensive professional franchises do not place more emphasis upon preseason and continuing psychological and psychiatric testing, interviewing and counseling. While from a humanitarian viewpoint, it is also incomprehensible why communities and school districts do not provide similar services for the young men and women they similarly expose to the stress of emotionally taxing athletic competition.

It is with this general background and orientation in mind that the following models were formulated. These plans, to my knowledge at the time of this writing, have not been attempted in *any* community or league in any part of the country. At the same time it is believed that their formulation and implementation will exert a positive effect upon the face of athletics turned toward the public, as well as upon the emotional health and performance of the participants.

The Team Psychologist-Psychiatrist

It is obvious that the most desirable method of dealing with emotional health of athletes is to employ a full- or part-time psychological or psychiatric consultant. This individual should be familiar with the sport, and be thoroughly trained in all aspects of clinical counseling. At the present time programs for the Ph.D. in sports psychology are beginning to appear within several university curriculums in the United States (including UCLA). Hopefully highly qualified people will be emerging from those.

This team consultant should be available during some of the team practices as is customary with regard to the team physician. He or she should also be on hand during games and be available for pre- and/or post-game counseling. His duties might also extend to psychological testing, counseling of coaches and of associated personnel as well as of team members.

At the same time, the institution of a team psychologist-psychiatrist at the professional level is fraught with problems. As has been pointed out by Scott,[6] among other writers, players will probably have a difficult time trusting such an individual. They will ask themselves, "Whose man is he, ours or management's?" They will probably carefully test him to ascertain the confidentiality of the material he will obtain, and whether he will use it for their well being or against them by exposing their psychic weaknesses to management at contract time? At the same time management is likely to be similarly suspicious of his presence, motives and operations. Is he likely to undermine the authority of the owners or coaches? they will ask themselves. Indeed the management of one professional team to whom the plan of a team psychological counselor was suggested refused to permit its institution because the psychologist would take the airplane seat of one of the many sportswriters who usually accompanied the team!

Such an individual may be impossible to find, for he must be interested in athletics but not too interested. He should be concerned about the mental health of the players, but not with his personal exposure in the press. Players would want his help, but would not want to read in the newspapers the day after a game that he is a primary source of their support and an integral part of their winning. The psychologist who goes on an "ego trip" is likely to render himself quickly ineffectual.

Athlete-Counselors

Professional teams invariably contain formal and informal counselors and leaders whom players confide in and go to in time of indecision and stress. At times these individuals acquire formal titles, "team representative" and the like. This player-counselor usually enjoys good rapport with fellow players, is respected and enjoys the confidence of a large number of peers.

One suggestion for imparting good psychological advice to members of athletic teams is to employ this team leader in a more formal counseling capacity. This team "rep" may be exposed to workshops lasting two to three days, once a year, in which the tools of the clinical counselor are explained and in which he learns how to deal with less serious problems, while acquiring the insights necessary to identify more pronounced signs of emotional disturbance which indicate the necessity for counseling and treatment by a back-up pool of professionals. This back-up team composed of clinical psychologists and/or psychiatrists, might be located in a central part of the country and called upon (flown in) when their services are obviously needed.

This type of model has been espoused by Arnold Beisser and others for use within contexts other than the athletic team. I believe, however, that it represents one of the most viable plans for use within professional athletic teams as they are now constituted in the United States.

The workshops would, of course, be conducted by the corps of professionals alluded to previously. These could be conducted yearly and run concurrently with regular meetings of the team representatives. The difficulty with this plan, as with the previously presented one, is the fact that various sports seasons run for different durations during the year, while problems needing attention may occur throughout the entire calendar year. Thus, part of the year the player might avail himself of the services of the professional corps described previously.

Institution Sports Council for Sport Sciences

Most colleges and universities presently contain various kinds of athletic policy boards, composed of interested professors, the athletic director, a coach or two, and members of the administration. The primary function, however, if one is to believe the minutes from their meetings, is to formulate athletic policies relative to finances, facilities and the procurement of athletes. Less often do their conversations turn to the physical and emotional protection of athletes once acquired.

It would seem helpful, and even moral, if universities and colleges also constitute a sports council composed of professionals on the campus (the school physician, psychologists, sociologists, etc. might be appropriate members) whose main concerns center upon the well-being of the athlete. These counsels might not only recommend policies which would implement the mental health of athletes, in the form of preventative psychiatry, but would also help in the improvement of performance standards. At the present time relationships between the athletic departments and schools and departments containing professionals who might aid athletes in rather direct ways are often informal and superficial. A council of the nature described could assist a productive wedding of sport, science, medicine and psychology and promote practices helpful to all concerned.

Community Sports Council

If community leaders, even within moderate-size cities, were to total up the number of people, children and adults, within their confines who participate in organized sport each year, they might be surprised at the number compiled. It would seem helpful if communities of 6,000 or more were to form what might be termed "sports councils." This council could be made up of interested and capable professional and lay individuals; people who are not only interested in sport, but who rate the interests of participants paramount. Such a council should contain at least one representative from the mental health professions, but need not be confined to this type of professional. Included also should be physicians, (orthopaedists, pediatricians, cardiologists and psychiatrists would seem most appropriate), educators, child development experts, psychiatric social workers, etc.

Such a group, meeting regularly, could formulate and implement policies which would not only include provisions for the protection of the mental and emotional health of sports participants within the community, but could also exert influence over the nature of insurance protection available; the formulation of standards for adequate facilities, training of officials, and the certification of coaches at all levels; and the institution of regular workshops available to parents, coaches, trainers and interested workers which would cover such subjects as the prevention, care and treatment of athletic injuries, coaching techniques, mental health aspects of sports participation, skill acquisition, developmental aspects of sports participation, and the influence of sports upon adults and upon the aged. This type of council could of course coordinate the efforts of the city government, local school districts, recreation programs, private and public athletic programs for youth, adults and the aged, and amateur athletic organizations. Personnel could be appointed and programs arranged which would provide for adequate emotional-health services for the sports participants within the boundaries of the city in which they are instituted.

The School Psychologist

There is hardly a school district of even moderate size in the United States that does not employ at least one school psychologist. This individual or group (numbering from 70–80 in several of the larger cities in the nation) generally possesses at least master's degree in clinical psychology. Duties include the counseling of parents and children with educational and/or emotional problems, the administration and interpretation of standard tests covering school achievement, intelligence, vocational aptitude and personality, as well as general consultation in curriculum and related matters.

The group provides an easily accessible and reasonably well-trained staff within a school district, which has at least an ancillary relationship to the school athletic program. One or several of these individuals should be permitted some time in their schedules each week, and during each school year, to aid in the maintenance of good mental health among the athletes within the school's jurisdiction.* For a school district to confine its attention only to the physical needs of its athletes by providing training room facilities and a consulting physician, without concomitant mental health services, is as short-sighted as similar practices among the large professional organizations who periodically lose the services of extremely high-priced athletes because of various kinds of mental and emotional breakdowns.

The local board of education, I believe, is morally responsible for the mental health of a youngster within their purview if at least part of his or her problems have stemmed from the accompanying stresses inherent in a program of interscholastic athletics. I believe that this responsibility might well be met through the use of the school psychologist(s) who might be engaged in several activities during a typical sports season including the following: (a) pre-season counseling of coaches and a meeting of the potential athletes describing the role of the psychologist and associated services; (b) the administration of sensitive and valid psychological instruments; (c) availability for personal counseling on the part of youngsters who might use their services; (d) attendance at a number of team practices and games; (e) follow-up and referral functions for youngsters who leave the district and who may need further work with a private psychiatrist or psychologist; (f) parent counseling, outlining the nature of emotional stresses to be placed on their youngsters, how the parent might assist in preventive mental health practices and how the parents' behavior and attitudes may add to or detract from the youngster's emotional health during a sports season.

Summary

It has been suggested that several types of models might aid in the maintenance of the mental health of athletes. These models are relatively specific to the various levels of athletics discussed, i.e. professional athletics, interschool competition and pre-high school competition. These models are as follows.

---

* It should be emphasized that I am suggesting paid time as part of their regular duties, not an unpaid extra.

Level	Suggested Model
Professional Athletics	Team psychiatrist-psychologist; or the use of team consultants trained to deal with immediate problems and to properly refer the more seriously disturbed teammate to a backup professional corps.
Collegiate-University Sports	Institutional Sports Council responsible for mental health protection and functions within the confines of the college or university.
Interscholastic Athletics	The use of the school psychologist to perform traditional counseling functions, testing, referral during and following a sports season.
Little League type of organization	Community Sports Council whose membership should include professional(s) conversant with mental health practices and who would implement helpful operations directly impinging upon coaches and their young athletes.

There are principles and questions ignored within the preceding paragraphs, including the nature of mental health counseling and services for female participants who are increasingly placed within stressful competitive situations. Likewise the thorny question of "whose man is he?" with regard to payment and responsibility within the professional organization was skirted. At the same time the procedures and principles when modified to suit specific situations, school districts, and communities should have a positive effect upon athletics, athletes, their coaches and their concerned parents.

BIBLIOGRAPHY

1. Beisser, Arnold: *The Madness in Sport.* New York, Appleton, 1967.
2. Cratty, B. J.: *Psychology in Contemporary Sport.* Englewood Cliffs, P-H, 1973.
3. ————: *Children and Youth in Competitive Sport: Guidelines for Parents and Coaches.* Freeport Long Island, Educational Activities Inc., 1974.
4. Frost, Reuben: *Psychological Concepts Applied to Physical Education and Coaching.* Reading, A-W, 1973.
5. Orlick, Terrance D.: Children sport: A revolution is coming. *J Can Assoc Health Phys Educ Recreation.*
6. Scott, Jac: *Athletics for Athletes.* Hayward, Other Way Book Co., 1968.
7. Skubic, Elvera: Studies of little league and middle league baseball. *Res Q,* 27:97–110, 1956.

PART V

SUMMARIES OF SELECTED
RESEARCH STUDIES

CHAPTER 20

DYNAMIC VISUAL ACUITY:
A DEVELOPMENTAL STUDY*

Introduction and Purpose

It has been only since World War II that researchers in various parts of the world have shown concern about the visual and visual-perceptual abilities required when dealing with the high velocities inherent in many sports activities.† In the 1950's, the review of the Russian studies by Graybiel [10] as well as investigations by Johannson in Sweden [13] and Hubbard and Senge [12] began to ignite minimal interest in the topic which was in turn reflected in what, for the most part, were piecemeal efforts.

For the most part only slight differences in various ocular characteristics were found when comparing athletes to non-athletes in some investigations, while the data from numerous other studies revealed no significant differences between athletes and nonathletes or between athletes in various sports.[4] One of the most comprehensive and cogent reviews of the topic is by Sanderson from Leeds University.[15]

Relevant to the topic of ocular and visual-perceptual characteristics in superior athletes is information from work on the development of similar characteristics in infants and children.

* Prepared for presentation at the 3rd International Congress for Psychology in Sport, Madrid, Spain, June 25–29, 1973. A complete monograph containing detailed procedures and findings may be obtained from the author at the University of California, Los Angeles. The study was supported in part by a Faculty Research Grant and through the cooperation of the Institute of Transportation and Traffic Engineering at UCLA and of Dr. Albert Burg, Research Psychologist for the Institute.

† An exception is a 1931 study by Bannister and Blackburn dealing with interpupillary distance in athletes.

Findings from the now classic "visual cliff" studies by Gibson and Walk,[9] the investigations of visual attention by Fantz and of visual judgments by Bower as well as investigations by Haith [11] and others reveal that the infant and the young child are capable of a wider variety of sophisticated visual behaviors and perceptual judgments than was once believed possible. The factor analysis by Smith and Smith published in 1966 [16] reveals that by five years of age the maturing visual-perceptual behaviors may be factored into at least five distinct abilities, a factor structure similar to that obtained from testing adult subjects.

Largely absent in the developmental literature are studies about two important aspects of visual behavior, (a) the accuracy with which children of various ages can anticipate future location(s) of moving objects, sometimes termed "perceptual anticipation" and (b) the degree to which children and youth at various ages are able to visually "stop" and select details from moving stimuli. This latter quality, referred to as dynamic visual acuity (DVA), is the focus of the investigation to be reported.[*,14]

Essentially the ability to extract detail from moving stimuli seems to rest upon at least four subabilities including (a) the ability to coordinate head with eye movement, (b) the ability to anticipate where a moving object will be so that it may be stopped for inspection, (c) ocular-motor coordination, and finally (d) the maturation of both the slow and the quick phases of what has been termed the optokinetic nystagmus reflex, one of the more basic and phylogenetically primitive orienting responses. This latter quality is functionally an attempt to keep a stable image on the retina for as long as possible during the movement of a stimulus through a field of vision.

Previous studies in which dynamic visual acuity has been investigated have employed adolescents and adults as subjects and a primary focus of these studies has been upon applied problems related to auto driving competencies.[3,14] Moreover, previous developmental studies of perceptual anticipation fre-

---

* A thorough literature review may be found in the monograph undergirding this presentation and in the chapter titled "Visual Perceptual Development" in B. J. Cratty, *Perceptual and Motor Development of Infants and Children* (New York, Macmillan, 1970).

quently required an accurate motor response from the subjects, thus rendering difficult the task of deciding whether the final results were influenced by motor or visual-perceptual competencies.[17,18]

It was thus purposed in this investigation to investigate dynamic visual acuity in children ranging in age from five to twelve years. Not only were age differences surveyed, but also differences in dynamic visual acuity which might be related to sex, race, and to selected ocular-visual characteristics including eye-color, eye-preference and whether or not the child wore corrective lenses.

Methods and Procedures

Four hundred seventy-five children (238 males and 237 females) from five to twelve years of age were tested in one measure of static acuity and three measures of dynamic visual acuity. The average age of the children was 8.41 years and 425 were Caucasian, thirty-eight Negro and twelve Oriental. Their I.Q.s averaged 112.

The apparatus has been employed in previous investigations by Burg and his colleagues and consists of a 35-mm slide projector mounted on a rotating cradle powered by a variable speed drive motor. The projector projects an acuity target (the Bausch and Lomb Ortho-Rater Acuity test checkerboard target) on a horizontally placed cylindrical screen, 180 degrees in extent with a four-foot radius. The screen is white, illuminated at approximately 7.8 footcandles with a 50 per cent reflecting factor. The entire apparatus was housed in a large trailer.

The subject sits in a chair with an adjustable height so that the pivot point of the projector cradle, the focal point of the projector, the center of the curvature of the screen and the center of the subject's head are all in vertical alignment. The projector causes two sets of fifteen slides, of decreasing sizes, to travel in a horizontal path across the screen from left to right.

Fifteen slides in set 1 were first presented statically with the projector immobile, with the subject asked to determine whether the checkerboard pattern was up, down, left or right. The fifteen slides in the second set were next presented moving at 60°/

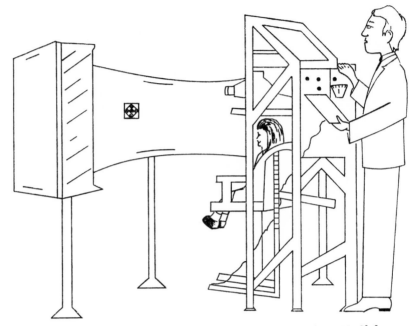

Figure 5. Apparatus to measure DYNAMIC VISUAL ACUITY. Slide projector directly over child's head rotates targets at various speeds.

second. Then the first set were shown again at 90°/second while after a two-minute rest period the second set were again shown one at a time at 120°/second.

During an orientation period the young subjects were acquainted with the nature of the target, shown manually how it moved and helped to say and indicate with the hand in which direction the checkerboard moved. During this period eye-preference was determined (via a one-eyed preferred sighting task) and eye-color was noted, together with information concerning race and whether or not corrective lenses were employed.

The visual angle formed by the slides ranged from the largest subtending ten minutes of arc to the smallest of .67 minutes of arc. These extremes corresponded to a Snellen rating of approximately 20/200 and 20/13 respectively.

The score employed was the slide last reported correctly by the subject in each series (static and at target speeds of 60, 90, and 120 degrees a second) after incorrectly responding on two slides consecutively.

Findings

1. Intercorrelations revealed higher generality of visual functioning in the children tested than was seen in previous studies using adult subjects. There were higher correlations between the tests of static acuity and dynamic acuity in children than in adults.

2. There was the expected drop-off effect as target speed became faster. However, the apparatus did not permit keeping constant intertrial times as target speeds increased and as the projector rotated at a constant speed.

3. One-way ANOVA revealed significant age differences at all target speeds with the most pronounced differences at the faster target speeds. (F scores ranged from 5.59 based upon scores of static acuity, to scores of 5.07, 4.25 and 9.54 under DVA conditions of 60°/second, 90°/second and 120°/second respectively.

4. It was apparent that approximately three levels of visual functioning were identifiable as a function of age, the first plateau from five to six years of age, a leveling off again from seven to nine years of age and a final level from ten to twelve years of age.

5. There were significant sex differences in the scores under all four visual conditions, as was found in previous studies.[3] F scores ranged from 13.6 (static acuity) and 16.6, 7.65 and 9.15 under DVA conditions of 60, 90, and 120 degrees per second target speed. The boys tested were superior under all four conditions.

6. There were no significant racial differences nor did classification of the subjects by eye preference reveal any differences in DVA or in static acuity.

7. Minor differences based upon eye color were noted at the faster target speeds. Blue-eyed children were significantly better than both hazel and green-eyed children at the fastest target speed (120°/sec).

8. Children who did not wear glasses were significantly superior to those who did, at all target speeds and under conditions evaluating static acuity.

It was thus concluded that significant age and sex differences did exist in the measures of static and dynamic acuity employed in this investigation. Other findings relative to ocular characteristics, it is believed, need more detailed inspection before any concrete conclusions may be drawn.

Implications and Recommendations

Further studies in this series will focus upon relationships between measures of DVA and sports skills, scores reflecting accurate perceptual anticipation as well as other measures of visual functioning.

Further investigation of the possible reasons underlying the sex differences and age differences found in this and in previous studies could revolve around experimental variables and around measures of neurological functioning and maturity.

BIBLIOGRAPHY

1. Bannister, H. and Blackburn, J. D.: An eye factor affecting proficiency at ball games. *Br J Psychol, 21*:382–384, 1931.
2. Bower, T. G.: The visual world of infants. *Sci Am, 215*:80–97, 1966.
3. Burg, Albert and Hulbert, S.: Dynamic visual acuity as related to age, sex and static acuity. *J Appl Psychol, 45*:111–116, 1961.
4. Cratty, B. J.: Visual-Space Perception. In *Movement Behavior and Motor Learning*. Philadelphia, Lea & Febiger, 1967, ch. 6.
5. ———: Visual Perceptual Development. In *Perceptual and Motor Development of Infants and Children*. New York, Macmillan, 1970, ch. 4.
6. ———. Apitzsch, E. and Bergel, R.: *Dynamic Visual Acuity: A Developmental Study*. Unpublished monograph, Los Angeles, Perceptual Motor Learning Laboratory, University of California, 1973.
7. Dayton, G. O., Jones, M. H., Steele, B. and Rose, M.: Developmental study of coordinated eye movements in the human infant. II. An electro-oculographic study of the fixation reflex in the newborn. *Arch. Ophthalmol, 71*:870–875, 1964.
8. Fantz, R. L.: Pattern vision in newborn infants. *Science, 140*:296–97, 1963.
9. Gibson, R. J. and Walk, R. D.: The visual cliff. *Sci Am, 4*:67–71, 1960.

10. Graybiel, A., Jokl, E. and Trapp, C.: Russian studies of vision in relation to physical activity and sports. *Res Q, 26:*480–485, 1955.

11. Haith, M. M.: The response of the human newborn to visual movement. *J Exp Child Psychol, 3:*235–243, 1966.

12. Hubbard, F. and Seng, C. N.: Visual movements of batters. *Res Q, 25:*42–57, 1954.

13. Johannson, G.: *Configurations in Event Perception.* Uppsala, Sweden, unpublished monograph, 1950.

14. Ludvigh, B. and Miller, J. W.: An analysis of dynamic visual acuity in a population of 200 naval aviation cadets. Pensacola, Jt. Proj. Rep. No. NM 001 075.01.07, USN Sch. Av. Medicine, 1954.

15. Sanderson, F. H.: Dynamic visual acuity and ball-game ability. Unpublished paper, Leeds, England, Leeds University, 1970.

16. Smith, O. W. and Smith, P. C.: Developmental studies of spatial judgments of children and adults. *Percept Mot Skills, 22:*57–156, monograph supplement, no. 1, 1966.

17. Whiting, H. T. A.: *Acquiring Ball Skill: A Psychological Interpretation.* London, G. Bell and Sons, 1969.

18. Williams, H. G.: The perception of moving objects by children. Unpublished study, UCLA Perceptual Learning Laboratory, 1967.

A COMPARISON OF MOVEMENT ATTRIBUTES EXHIBITED BY CHICANO, ANGLO AND BLACK CHILDREN*

Introduction

COMPARATIVE STUDIES contrasting the abilities of black and white children have, with few exceptions been limited to performance on intellectual tests and performances in educational settings.[2]

The few studies which have been conducted comparing the motor abilities of white and black children have produced findings which suggest that the young black child can run faster than the young white child of both sexes,[3] while in another instance it was found that young black children were more likely to be able to replicate a complicated rhythmic pattern, than were his white counterparts.[6]

This present study was conducted to determine if there were significant differences in the manner in which Anglo, black and Chicano children perform in selected movement tasks. In contrast to previous studies dealing with this same topic, a wider variety of motor tasks has been employed in this study. In addition to measures of running speed and endurance, throwing, strength and balance tasks, as well as a measure of self-control were employed.

---

* Study carried out in Santa Monica, California by Robert Bonds with the co-operation of the Santa Monica City Schools and the Perceptual-Motor Learning Laboratory, UCLA. This summary was prepared by B. J. Cratty, Director of the Laboratory.

Methods and Procedures

Three groups of five-year-old males were selected for the study, enrolled in kindergarten classes within the Santa Monica city schools—thirty from each of the racial-ethnic subgroups. None of the ninety subjects, at the time of the testing had reached his sixth birthday. Three testers assessed the children individually, and the testers were in racial and ethnic subgroups similar to those of the children each one tested.

Five types of tests were employed: a test of running speed (30 yards), a test of running-walking endurance (440 yards which the child could either walk, run, or engage in some combination of both), a test of grip strength, a self-control test ("How slowly can you walk this 12-foot long line?"), and three tests of static balance, each of which had to be maintained under control for at least five seconds on a pass-fail basis (one with feet together and parallel, a one-foot balance, and a third in which a heel-toe position had to be maintained). The final test administered was a softball throw for distance.

Findings

Intergroup comparisons revealed the following:

1. The black children were significantly stronger in the hand-grip measures than were Anglo and Chicano children. No significant differences were found between Chicano and white Anglo children in this measure.

2. Black children were significantly faster in the thirty-yard run, than were the Chicano and Anglo children. Again there were no significant differences between the latter two groups.

3. Black children were able to throw a softball significantly farther than were both the Anglo and Chicano groups. No significant differences were seen between the throwing efforts of the white Anglo and Chicano youngsters.

4. The Chicano children evidenced significantly less impulse control in the "how slowly can you walk" test than did the black, and white Anglo youngsters. No differences in this measure were recorded when the scores of the latter groups were contrasted.

5. Although statistically no significant intergroup differences

were found when the scores collected in the quarter mile walk-run test were compared, the mean scores of the white Anglo youngsters were slower by 152.6 seconds than the mean scores of both the Chicano (138.9 secs) and black younsters (135.4 secs).

6. A significantly greater percentage of the black youngsters (86%) passed the heel-toe stand test of static balance than was evidenced by the white Anglo boys (60% passed) and the Chicano males (60%).

It was therefore concluded that, based upon the limited sampling tested that the black youngsters were significantly stronger in grip-strength, ran significantly faster, evidenced better balance ability and threw farther than did the two other racial-ethnic subgroups evaluated.

Discussion

These findings generally support those collected previously by Hutinger regarding the superiority of running speed of young black youngsters.[3] The findings that the black children were stronger and evidenced better balance also suggest that future studies with a larger and more representative sampling should explore possible inherent maturational reasons for these differences as well as differences in childrearing practices and in general social expectations which could account for the possible superiority of black children in these measures.

The findings that Chicano youngsters performed less well than did the other groups in the tests of impulse control might also be delved into more thoroughly, correlating such measures and findings to teachers' reports of classroom conformity as well as to other measures of academic achievement. The lack of significant differences between the black children and the Anglo children in this measure of impulse control is not in agreement with the findings of a previous study by Burke[1]—a further indication that more work is needed concerning this potentially useful measure.

The relatively young age, five years, of the subjects leads one to believe that the total school experience may have relatively little direct effect upon the superior motor abilities often seen in later life on the part of black athletes. Apparently black youngsters, if the findings of this study are considered valid, enter school with certain abilities superior to their white Anglo and Chicano peers. Thus further efforts should be focused upon the potentially useful but elusive questions surrounding whether black children and youth are inherently superior in motor ability and/or whether later superiority seen in the incidence of black athletes on professional teams is the result of not only an early good start in physical activities, but also is dependent upon the ways in which the culture shapes and rewards them for displaying their physical prowess.

BIBLIOGRAPHY

1. Burke, K.: A Survey of Selected Self-Control Measures in Elementary School Children. Unpublished Study, Perceptual-Motor Learning Laboratory, UCLA, 1970.
2. Dreger, R. M. and Miller, K. S.: Comparative psychological studies of Negroes and whites in the United States: 1959–1965. *Psychol Bull Monogr Supplement*, 1968, vol. 70 (3, Pt. 2).
3. Hutinger, P. W. "Differences in speed between American Negro and white children in performance of the 35-yard dash." *Res Q, 30:* 366–368, 1959.
4. Metheny, E.: Some differences in bodily proportions between American Negro and white, male college students, as related to athletic performance. *Res Q, 10:*41, 1939.
5. Rhodes, A.: A comparative study of motor abilities of Negroes and whites. *Child Dev,* 8:369–371, 1937.
6. Van Alstyne, D. and Osborne, E.: Rhythmic responses of Negro and white children 2 to 6. *Monogr Soc Res Child Dev,* vol. 2, no. 4, serial no. 2, 1939.
7. Worthy, M. and Markle, A.: Racial differences in reactive versus self-paced sports activities. *J Pers Soc Psychol, 16:*439–443, no. 3, 1970.

THE EFFECTS OF LEARNING GAMES
UPON SELECTED ACADEMIC
ABILITIES OF BLACK AND
MEXICAN-AMERICAN CHILDREN
WITH LEARNING PROBLEMS*

I N MEASURES OF ATTENTION and task persistence the children
exposed to learning games evidenced significantly more improvement than did the children in the group afforded special
small-group classroom tutoring. (I.e. in a line-walking task, such
as "walk a 12′ line as slowly as you can," the final means were
42 seconds for the learning games group, and 26 seconds for the
classroom tutoring group. Both group means were about 15
seconds in preliminary teaching.)

2. The final scores in letter recognition (i.e. the ability to re-
cite the alphabet in correct order): the learning games group
performed significantly better (at the 1% level) than did the
classroom tutoring group (22 letters correct to over 25 letters
correct as mean scores).

3. In all the measures of serial memory (i.e. remembering
letters, numbers, and pictures in order) when given orally or
presented visually, the learning games group evidenced significantly more improvement and achieved significantly higher

---

* Findings from a Research Study sponsored by the U.S. Department of Education, Bureau of Handicapped Children, carried out in Los Angeles, within six
schools in the Catholic Archdiocese, from 1968 to 1970. (Detailed findings are
available in monograph form, Department of Kinesiology, UCLA.)

scores than did the groups exposed to special classroom tutoring.

4. By midway through the first semester, 75 per cent of the first graders in the learning games group evidenced the ability to identify all letters of the alphabet perfectly while only 30 per cent of the children in the special classroom tutoring in small groups were able to do so.

5. The children in the learning games group evidenced significantly higher spelling scores (at the 1% level) than did the children exposed to special classroom tutoring. There were thirteen out of twenty words correct as compared to nine correct words posted by the children given special classroom tutoring.

6. In all three measures of serial memory ability the learning games group evidenced significant improvement (at the 1% and 5% levels), while the children in the special tutoring groups did not evidence any significant improvement in any of the three serial memory tasks.

7. In a total score derived from combining scores of balance and two scores of agility, both the learning games group and the special classroom tutoring group initially posted scores of eighteen; in the final testing the learning games group registered improvement in this combined score which was significantly better (at the 1% level) than the final average score of the children exposed to classroom tutoring.

ANNOTATED BIBLIOGRAPHY

Books

A. FOR PHYSICAL EDUCATORS

1. *Movement Behavior and Motor Learning*, Philadelphia, Lea & Febiger, 1974 (3rd ed.)

   A graduate and upper division text outlining and interpreting research findings dealing with motor learning and performance. Chapters include those dealing with movement and communication, neurological bases of learning and performance, evolution of human movement, motivation, social motives, maturation, transfer of training and the influences of selected practice factors. The bibliography contains 1400 references.

2. *Social Dimensions of Physical Activity.* Englewood Cliffs, P-H, 1967.

   A review of the literature dealing with the manner in which social factors influence the motor performance of individuals. Chapters include those dealing with the influence of the family, the audience, personality-physique relationships, and the like. Contains a 500-item bibliography.

3. *Psychology and Physical Activity.* Englewood Cliffs, P-H, 1968.

   A simple and direct outline of research findings and their practical implications for teachers of physical education and coaches. Contains chapters on the clumsy child and the superior athlete, as well as sections on motivation, motor learning, perception, social factors, and the like.

4. *New Perspectives of Man in Action.* With Roscoe Brown, Ed.D., Englewood Cliffs, P-H, 1969.

5. *Experiments in Motor Performance and Motor Learning.* With Robert Hutton, Philadelphia, Lea & Febiger, 1969.

   Contains twenty-five laboratory experiences for physical

educators taking courses in motor learning and/or the psychology of physical activity. Research requires little in the way of equipment and at the same time suggestions for additional research are included.

6. *Psychology and the Superior Athlete.* With Dr. Miroslav Vanek (Charles University, Prague, Czechoslovakia), New York, Macmillan, 1969.

A text outlining research and practical implications derived from over fifty years study of athletes in Russia and the Eastern countries, as well as in other parts of the world. Particularly interesting should be chapters on the history of sports psychology, as well as sections dealing with the testing and clinical aspects of sports psychology carried out with the Czech teams during the 1968 Olympics. Case studies conclude this book.

7. *Movement Activities, Motor Ability and the Education of Children.* With M. M. Martin, C. Jennett, M. Ikeda and M. Morris, Springfield, Thomas, 1970.

A summary of research carried out by post-doctoral students in 1968 under the supervision of Dr. Bryant J. Cratty. Studies dealing with the self-concept, changes in motor performance with training, the uses of learning games to change academic competencies, and the game choices and self-concept of clumsy youngsters are contained in the book.

8. *Career Potentials of Physical Activity.* Englewood Cliffs, P-H, 1971.

A thorough coverage of over fourteen careers which a student might choose dealing with physical activity, as well as numerous chapters concerning the content of curriculum suited to these careers. Intended for physical education major students, and those in similar service majors.

9. *Physical Expressions of Intelligence.* Englewood Cliffs, P-H, 1972.

A thorough review of research and theories relating movement to intelligence. Chapters include a history of the concept of intelligence, intelligence testing, mental practice, theories linking movement to learning, academic improvement, language learning through movement, and the like.

Contains practical examples, as well as the rationale upon which movement education and physical education programs may be based.

10. *Psychology in Contemporary Sport.* Englewood Cliffs, P-H, 1973.

A comprehensive look at all aspects of psychology with relationship to coaching and performance in competitive athletics. Includes chapters on motivation, personality of athletes, social interactions on teams, leadership in sports, the personality of the coach, conducting team practices, and the teaching of motor skills.

11. *Teaching Motor Skills.* Englewood Cliffs, P-H, 1973.

A simply written monograph outlining how one may teach motor skills effectively. Material is accompanied by diagrams and bibliographies, as well as by summaries on such topics as motivation, practice conditions, motivation, retention of skill, and the use of instruction to encourage optimum learning and retention.

See also numbers B2, B5, B10, C1, C2, C4, C5.

B. FOR SPECIAL EDUCATORS AND PARENTS OF ATYPICAL CHILDREN

1. *Developmental Sequences of Perceptual-Motor Tasks for Neurologically Handicapped and Retarded Children.* Freeport, Long Island, Educational Activities, 1967.

A paperback outlining reasonable levels of difficulty in the motor education of atypical children. Chapters contain sequences dealing with body image, drawing and writing, balance, gross motor ability, strength and fitness, moving and thinking, catching, throwing balls, locomotion, and teaching guidelines.

2. *Moving and Learning: Fifty Games for Children with Learning Difficulties.* Freeport Long Island, Educational Activities, 1968.

A card film of fifty games including those enhancing motor abilities as well as those leading toward academic competencies, including spelling, mathematics, and the like.

3. *Developmental Games for Physically Handicapped Children.* Palo Alto, Peek Publications, 1969.

An illustrated monograph of games for physically handicapped children to enhance movement abilities, as well as academic and perceptual abilities, includes sections on sensory-motor stories ("Johnny, Bunny and Goose!"), wheel chair games, and also contains specific suggestions for equipment modifications to accommodate physically handicapped youngsters.

4. *Motor Activities and the Education of Retardates.* Philadelphia, Lea & Febiger, 1969.

Contains theoretical, as well as practical guidelines for the uses of movement in the education of retarded children. Chapters dealing with the principles of learning skills, as well as illustrated chapters containing suggestions for the improvement of handwriting, big muscle coordination, and the like are contained in the text, together with a section on the self-concept. The appendix contains a screening test, together with averages which may be applied to retarded youngsters.

5. *Physical Development for Children.* Freeport Long Island, Educational Activities, 1973. Two hundred five game and activity cards for the normal and atypical child.

6. *Perceptual-Motor Efficiency in Children: The Measurement and Improvement of Movement Attributes.* With Sister Margaret Mary Martin. Philadelphia, Lea & Febiger, 1969.

A book devoted to explaining why and how children with coordination problems may be aided. Chapters dealing with the control of large muscle activity, evaluation and norms, principles of perceptual-motor training, handwriting activity, and the like are contained in this well illustrated text.

7. *Perceptual-Motor Behavior and Educational Processes.* Springfield, Thomas, 1969.

A text containing speeches given by Dr. Cratty from 1965 to 1968, dealing with perceptual-motor functioning and the uses of movement with various types of atypical children, including the blind, the retarded, the neurologically impaired, and the physically handicapped. The appendix of the text contains a screening test for use with the blind, as well as a test of motor proficiency.

8. *Trampoline Activities for Atypical Children.* Palo Alto, Peek Publications, 1969.

    A monograph, illustrated, containing guidelines for the use of the trampoline as a developmental tool. Sections on conditioning exercises, safety hints, as well as balance, body image, and agility training add to the book.

9. *Movement and Spatial Awareness in Blind Children and Youth.* Springfield, Thomas, 1971.

    A comprehensive practicum of activities, as well as a theoretical review of research dealing with the manner in which blind infants, children, and youth learn about space through movement and through interpreting auditory experiences. Chapters include body-image development in the blind, auditory perception, object detection, map reading, assessing motor abilities, improving motor abilities, and the like. Research from all over the world is employed as a basis for the content.

10. *Active Learning.* Englewood Cliffs, P-H, 1971.

    A beautifully illustrated paperback containing over 100 learning games intended to enhance a variety of academic abilities including reading, mathematics, memory letter recognition, and the like. Sections on impulse control and improving motor ability and fitness are also contained in this book. Research upon which the games have been based was carried out within the central city of Los Angeles from 1967 to 1971.

11. *Teaching About Human Behavior Through Active Games.* Englewood Cliffs, P-H, 1974.

    This forward-looking monograph contains numerous practical activities and vigorous games intending to enhance language abilities, reading and prereading competencies, memorization, categorization, evaluation, as well as such problem-solving abilities as analysis, synthesis, divergent thinking, convergent thinking, and reversibility and flexibility of problem solving operations. Appropriate for elementary school teachers, special education teachers and instructors of the gifted child.

See also numbers 7, 9, C1, C2, C3, C4, C5.

C. FOR ELEMENTARY EDUCATORS

1. *Movement, Perception, and Thought.* Palo Alto, Peek Publications, 1969.

   A monograph listing the stages through which children may be brought to elicit academic improvement through movement. This illustrated book contains sections on impulse control, mathematic games, spelling games, and the like.

2. *Perceptual and Motor Development of Infants and Children.* New York, Macmillan, 1970.

   A comprehensive paperback containing a thorough overview and interpretation of the research dealing with perceptual and motor functioning of infants and children; sections include infant reflexes, early motor development, social development in play, visual perceptual development, interpretation of perceptual-motor theories, as well as a concluding chapter presenting a theoretical model for the consideration of the maturation of human abilities.

3. *Sounds, Words, and Actions: 50 Movement Games to Enhance the Language Art Skills of Elementary School Children.* With Sister Mark Szczepanik. Freeport Long Island, Educational Activities, 1971.

   A package of game cards aiding in the teaching of letter sounds, spelling, and reading skills. Researched for four years in the central city of Los Angeles.

4. *Educational Activities for the Physically Handicapped.* With James S. Breen. Denver, Love Publishing Company, 1972.

   Numerous practical games are included in this well-illustrated text, games for the physically handicapped youngster on the playground. Lead-up activities, various table games, more vigorous games, as well as games tapping various academic and intellectual qualities are described.

5. *Physical Activities for Enhancing Intellectual Abilities.* Englewood Cliffs, P-H, 1973.

Clearly outlined are games which purportedly tap various intellectual abilities, including memorization, evaluation, categorization, and problem solving behaviors including convergent-divergent thinking, analysis and synthesis, flexibility and reversibility in problem solving. Other games are aligned with basic communicative abilities including expressive language and reading.

See also numbers 2, B1, B5, B6, B8, B10, B11, B12.

D. GENERAL

1. *Some Educational Implications of Movement Experiences.* Seattle, Spec Child, 1969.

    A text containing essays dealing with the manner in which movement experiences relate to various components of the educational processes.

2. *Human Behavior: Understanding Educational Processes.* Wolfe City, University Pr, 1971.

    A comprehensive text for students dealing with the psychology of the learning process. Chapters on language learning, perceptual learning, intelligence, creativity, social factors important in school, as well as sections on maturation, and the like are found in this text.

    See also numbers A4, A9, B7, B10, C1, C2, C5.

Research Monographs

1. *Perceptual Thresholds of Non-Visual Locomotion, Part I.* Sponsored by the National Institute of Neurological Diseases and Blindness, Washington, D.C., 1965.

2. *Perceptual Thresholds of Non-Visual Locomotion, Part II.* With Harriet Williams, sponsored by the National Institute of Neurological Diseases and Blindness, Washington, D.C., 1966.

3. *The Perceptual-Motor Attributes of Mentally Retarded Children and Youth.* Sponsored by the Mental Retardation Services Board, Los Angeles County, California, 1966.

4. *Figural After-Effects Elicited by Selected Bodily Movements.* With Kirt E. Duffy. Sponsored by the National Science Foundation, Washington, D.C., 1967.

5. *The Body Image of Blind Children.* With Theressa Sams,

International Research Information Service, American Foundation of the Blind, New York, 1969.

6. *Studies of Movement Aftereffects.* With Kirt E. Duffy, sponsored by the National Sciences Foundation, Washington, D.C., monograph supplement, *Percept Mot Skills*, 1969.

7. *The Effects of a Program of Learning Games Upon Selected Academic Abilities of Children with Learning Difficulties.* With Sister Margaret Mary Martin. Washington, D.C., Bureau of Education for the Handicapped, U.S. Office of Education, 1970.

8. *The Effects of a Program of Learning Games Upon Selected Academic Abilities of Children with Learning Difficulties.* With Sister Mark Szczepanik. Washington, D.C. Bureau of Education for the Handicapped, U.S. Office of Education, 1971.

9. *The Psychomotor Skills of Dental Trainees.* With Drs. Kenneth Trabert, D.D.S. and Eugene Hanson D.D.S., Center for the Health Sciences, UCLA, 1973, monograph.

10. *Dynamic Visual Acuity: A Developmental Study.* With Erwin Apitzsch, and Reinhard Bergel, Perceptual-Motor Learning Laboratory UCLA Monograph, 1974.

11. *The Special Olympics: A National Opinion Survey,* sponsored by the Joseph P. Kennedy Jr. Foundation, 1972, Monograph, Perceptual-Motor Learning Laboratory, UCLA.

INDEX

187